Standing Qigong *for* Health *and* Martial Arts

—————— ZHAN ZHUANG ——————

STANDING QIGONG
for Health *and* Martial Arts
—— ZHAN ZHUANG ——

Noel Plaugher

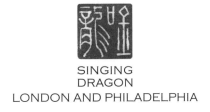

SINGING
DRAGON
LONDON AND PHILADELPHIA

First published in 2015
by Singing Dragon
an imprint of Jessica Kingsley Publishers
73 Collier Street
London N1 9BE, UK
and
400 Market Street, Suite 400
Philadelphia, PA 19106, USA

www.singingdragon.com

Library of Congress Cataloging in Publication Data
Plaugher, Noel.
  Standing Qigong for health and martial arts, Zhan Zhuang / Noel Plaugher.
    pages cm
  Includes index.
  ISBN 978-1-84819-257-7 (alk. paper)
  1. Qi gong--Health aspects. 2. Martial arts--Health aspects. I. Title. II. Title:
Standing Qi gong for health
and martial arts, Zhan Zhuang.
  RA781.8.P53 2015
  613.7'1489--dc23
                              2014047509

British Library Cataloguing in Publication Data
A CIP catalogue record for this book is available from the British Library

ISBN 978 1 84819 257 7
eISBN 978 0 85701 204 3

Printed and bound in the United States

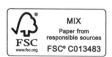

This book is dedicated both to my teachers and to my students. I have learned equally from them all.

CONTENTS

DISCLAIMER

Every effort has been made to ensure that the information contained in this book is correct, but it should not in any way be substituted for medical advice. Readers should always consult a qualified medical practitioner before adopting any complementary or alternative therapies. Neither the author nor the publisher takes responsibility for any consequences of any decision made as a result of the information contained in this book.

ACKNOWLEDGMENTS

I sincerely thank my wife Brenda and my son Christopher, who inspire me to strive for more, Sifu Johnny Jang for being a great teacher, Richard Trammell for being a great friend and mentor, and my friend Debbie Auerbach for the photography.

INTRODUCTION

I have been looking for a book that shows postures for standing Qigong for health and martial arts for some time. I have seen many books that talk about postures for health, but I have never seen one that included the many standing postures for martial arts as well. When I started studying internal martial arts, the first thing that attracted me was the standing postures and how they improved my health and increased martial power. I was amazed that so many styles of internal martial arts included standing as part of their power training. My aim with this book is to bring all of the health and martial postures together in one volume so that they can be easily referenced by all practitioners.

You have probably never heard of me, and you may not be familiar with standing Qigong. Let me tell you a little about both. First, about myself. I started studying martial arts in 1990 after being a victim of violent crime. That event was transformative for me and led me to martial arts and ultimately to *internal* martial arts and Qigong. I had no interest in martial arts prior to that time, and I was exposed to martial arts only through the martial arts films I grew up with. To me, martial arts was basically what I saw in those movies: guys flying around, making strange sounds, and doing physically dubious feats. All of the things associated with martial arts were to me unrealistic, antiquated, and weird, and they didn't really fit with the world as I knew it. It might as well have been voodoo, as it was potently alien to me, a kid from the suburbs in northern California. I figured martial arts was just some strange Asian stuff that people do out of tradition, but that there wasn't really anything to it, so I basically dismissed it all out of hand.

While recovering from my incident, I was persuaded by a friend to study martial arts to help work through my posttraumatic stress, anxiety, and also to gain confidence. I was dubious about how helpful it would be, and I had absolutely no aptitude for martial arts or most things physical. I didn't play sports, and frankly I wasn't interested in anything that involved sweating. My friend eventually won out, though, and drove me to class one night. I did indeed end up studying martial arts, and I struggled with it for a long time. It was not easy for me. In fact, it was the hardest thing I ever did. The concepts and techniques I became exposed to were very effective, though, especially the use of the mind. Often when my instructor would talk about "thinking" this or that for a desired effect, I would be surprised by the results— for example, the idea of thinking that my leg was like iron, and immovable, and could be used to kick out the opponent's leg. And then to test it and find that it actually worked! I was just amazed at the power of the mind and body working together. This was my first introduction to using the mind effectively, and it was my first experience with the mind's power over the body. I became very interested in how far this type of thinking could go and I wanted to learn more.

My teacher had told me that there was another branch of martial arts called *internal martial arts*. He told me that they focused more on the mind-body connection and intention, and that they were a great way to obtain internal power. This all sounded good to me and I filed away the names of these styles—Xing Yi Quan, Ba Gua Quan, and Tai Chi Quan—knowing that at some point I would seek them out.

In time, I achieved my goal of black belt and started thinking that this would be a good time to look into internal martial arts. Over the years of studying martial arts I definitely changed for the better. My body became healthy and I felt pretty good about myself. I am a very different person now from the person who started so long ago, and I attribute that growth to my teachers and the continued pursuit of knowledge. Martial arts, in all of its forms, has been an incredible learning experience, and I enjoy learning, teaching, and practicing all forms of martial arts styles to this day.

★

So what is standing Qigong? Standing Qigong (energy work) or Zhan Zhuang (post-standing) is a method of developing internal power and improving your overall health. Standing still in fixed postures is an internal and physical workout that will benefit your body and mind. You will be amazed at the amount of pleasant and satisfying work standing can be, and you will be more amazed at the results you can achieve both physically and mentally by simply standing.

You do not need to be a practitioner of a martial art to feel the benefits of standing Qigong. In fact, I first heard of standing Qigong from a friend who was prescribed "Holding the sphere below" (a health stance explained and demonstrated in Chapter 3) for his arthritis. He had been referred to a practitioner of Traditional Chinese Medicine (TCM) after having tried all the available treatments. I was pretty skeptical about the whole thing. Can standing in one spot really do anything? It seemed a little unusual to me, and I didn't really understand how it could work. I asked him about a month later if it was working, and he said it was. This really piqued my interest and I started investigating the internal side of martial arts.

Can standing achieve any measurable results? I was still a little doubtful, but I wanted to check it out. My first proper lesson in standing Qigong was when I asked a friend to refer me to a doctor who practiced TCM. I was told he practiced Tai Chi Quan and Qigong as well. I told him I was very interested in standing Qigong. He set up a time to come and learn how to stand. I brought along a couple of my intrepid friends who were also interested, and we joked that we would learn how to shoot lightning bolts out of our hands. We didn't expect much, but on we went anyway, eager to receive our first lesson.

After some brief pleasantries, the teacher walked us out to the front parking lot of his office, which was situated in a strip mall. I looked around a little confused. "Are we going to do it here?" I asked. The parking lot was pretty busy, and I was a little self-conscious about doing something which I thought of as private in such a public place. He assured me, "Don't worry, they won't bother us." I hadn't thought of it that way, but I liked the way the focus was taken from what others might think to what *we* think, and how it can't really affect us unless we let it.

We stood in a circle in front of his storefront and started with "holding the sphere." We were instructed to "just stand." He would check on us every once in a while and make minor alignment adjustments to our hands, hips, or head which were always followed by the reminder, "Relax." Eventually, as we stood for a while, I thought he must have lost track of time. *How long have we been out here?* I could feel that the shadows and sun had moved a bit. As cars passed I could hear them slow more than usual and I knew that they were probably watching, curious about these people standing in a circle with their hands held as if holding an imaginary beach ball. I tried to block it out and focus on what I was doing, not what others were possibly thinking, since in reality, I don't know what people are thinking.

As we stood there quietly, with only the sounds of footsteps, car doors opening and closing, and tires slowly creeping by, I became curious. What is the teacher doing? I peeked a bit and saw that the teacher was standing as we were. *How long has it been?* It seemed like a long time to stand still. My mind would run wild before finally returning to what I was doing. Eventually, he said, "Okay, go ahead and drop your arms, and shake out your legs." I was surprised that I was sweaty, and my muscles felt sore in some places, especially my legs and shoulders. I asked how long we had stood, and he said a half hour. I can tell you that is probably longer than I would advise a beginning student to try, but he also knew we were practicing a martial art, and I think he expected that we could handle a heavier dose the first time. Regardless, I felt it was challenging and completely different from anything that I had tried before. My body felt unified and more connected. That is not the best description, but it is the only one I can think of at the moment. My two friends thought that it was interesting and probably useful, but they weren't sure about embarking on studying. But I had made up *my* mind that I wanted to learn more.

I started with an experiment to really feel how I could cultivate more energy and power by standing in the "embrace the sphere" posture every day for about 15–20 minutes, for a month. I was instructed to either conduct my practice early or late to benefit the most from the change of day: night to day or day to night. By doing your practice in the early or late part of the day you are able to obtain the benefit of the change from yin to yang and yang to yin according to the theory of TCM. I don't think that this is necessary anymore, but it is a good guideline to keep your practice consistent and to make sure you can always fit it into your day.

I would rise early and stand using all of the directives given to me by my instructor. He told me to focus on the breath, relax, and use the images to keep the proper alignment. The first couple of days were a real challenge physically, but then it quickly became less of a physical challenge and more of a mental one. I found that my mind would wander as it had in the parking lot, thinking of work, conversations, that bill that needed to be paid, and so forth. But using the techniques I was given, I was able to bring my mind back to the "now." I didn't realize that I would essentially be meditating and exercising at the same time. I was really excited about this incredible dual-purpose exercise. I looked forward to this new practice every morning.

Within about a week or two, I was totally blown away by how I felt. I felt more power overall, and I felt really good. It is difficult to completely describe, but I felt solid, strong, full, and many other adjectives that don't really adequately describe something so amazing. The main thing was that I felt "something." I knew that there was something tangible to standing Qigong, and I really started to yearn to learn more. The two postures that I knew, so far, seemed really powerful, but I had heard about and read about more postures. This started me on an odyssey into studying standing Qigong, as well as the internal martial arts, that lasted years and continues to this day. Most importantly, I am glad I did it.

I started practicing standing to improve my martial arts and gain more internal power. I was pleasantly surprised to find out that my health improved as well. I felt better. I started to use visualization techniques as well. For example, when I am feeling a little ill, I can think of my body gaining energy from the earth or sky to pump up my energy and get me going onto a fast recovery. I want to be careful to not lead anyone to take my anecdotal experience as the norm, but I do want to express that I have felt better using standing Qigong. It has worked for me.

Through standing I felt the mind-body connection at a deeper level than before. I was able to see the results in my martial arts. My body felt stronger and more unified. Everything just seemed to go together better. My workout partners would also express how much stronger kicks and punches felt. I felt immovable and yet able to move through others. I felt stronger and I was using less effort. I just felt really good, but more importantly, I felt an overall sense of calm and positive energy.

This was all new to me, and I felt that I was really onto something. I couldn't believe who everyone doing martial arts wasn't supplementing their training with standing Qigong. I tried to tell a few people, but they seemed to dismiss it or think it was too much trouble. I couldn't believe it. For a while, I went on my own.

Eventually, I sought a teacher who could show me more about internal arts and standing Qigong specifically. I really wanted to explore the world of internal martial arts. I had certainly heard of Tai Chi Quan, but I wanted something more exotic. Granted there are many great forms of Tai Chi Quan, and some are very rare, but I still wanted something a little farther out. Ba Gua Quan was interesting, but I felt it didn't emphasize the standing enough, and I was really looking for something that incorporated standing. Eventually, I settled on Xing Yi Quan, which seemed interesting because of its simplicity of having just a few forms and the emphasis on standing in the San Ti Shi posture, which is the cornerstone of the style.

I checked out the internal art of Xing Yi Quan, and the more I discovered, the more I liked it. I was really attracted to the emphasis on generating energy, power, and incorporating your intention. There were just a few forms. There are the five elements—metal, water, fire, wood, and earth (I've included the Five Element Linking Form in this book)—and twelve animals. It seemed like a pretty "stripped down" style that emphasized some extremely simple, but powerful, concepts. It seemed the epitome of "less is more." The next step was to find a teacher.

Where was I going to find a Xing Yi Quan teacher? Of all of the internal arts I had to choose from, Xing Yi Quan was definitely the rarest. Although that actually appealed to me even more, it didn't change the fact that it would likely be difficult to find a teacher. At the time, I felt like I wanted to go far away from what I had been studying. I felt like I was going to learn something really unusual, and that was very attractive.

A friend told me that the best way to find out about a Chinese martial art in the San Francisco Bay Area is to go to Chinatown, where there are two Chinatown neighborhoods. The most famous is in San Francisco itself, which is a tourist destination. The other is in Oakland, across the Bay from San Francisco. Oakland Chinatown is less flashy, and I like it better for authenticity. The street signs are in Chinese, the people speak Chinese almost exclusively, and Chinese culture is prominent in the form of restaurants, Buddhist temples, and large, beautifully printed signs in Chinese characters. There is just a certain relaxed atmosphere that appealed to me and seemed unpretentious.

I arranged to meet my friend at a plaza downtown in the early hours of Sunday morning. As I drove to the heart of Chinatown, I saw the Buddhist temples being attended and I noticed that Chinese language signs were everywhere. As I got close to the location I could see the plaza. There were many large and small groups of people studying various things. This was definitely different from what I was used to. I walked from my car and I could smell incense coming from somewhere. It was pungent but not unpleasant. I saw people sitting in meditation in a circle by a large pillar, and then I walked past the pillar and saw the whole plaza. There were people grouped into various classes, and each had an instructor at the front of the group. There was a group of people close by studying Tai Chi Quan Sword being led by a woman who looked to be in her eighties. I watched for a moment and was amazed as she cross-stepped as deeply as anyone I had ever seen, and she did it with ease. I was more intrigued than ever to learn more.

I had been told to meet the teacher close by the entrance to the plaza. I saw him. He was a middle-aged Asian man dressed in a black shirt and Kung Fu pants. I was surprised he wasn't wearing the traditional shirt with the frog buttons, but I was pleased to see him dressed casually as it made me a bit more relaxed. I really didn't want to deal with the pomp and circumstance that can sometimes accompany, and be so dominant in, martial arts. I was immediately put at ease meeting my new teacher, Sifu Johnny Jang. He was really pleasant, with a big smile, and he seemed to be excited that I was interested in Xing Yi Quan. When I asked why he was happy about my studying Xing Yi Quan, he said, "It means I get to practice!" Like most great teachers, Sifu looked at teaching as a way to improve himself while imparting wisdom to his students. He had such a great attitude that I was really looking forward to learning from him.

He told me a little about Xing Yi Quan that I had not heard. I asked him why it is that so many people who study internal martial arts have studied Xing Yi Quan, and then they study something else. He said that Xing Yi Quan is usually taught first so the student can fight, but then the student sometimes gets bored with it and wants something with more material. I told him I had enough material, and I didn't want any more than was necessary. I was interested in substance. We started into the lesson right away. The first thing he showed me was how to stand in San Ti Shi. I had seen the posture before, but this was the first time I received any specific instruction regarding how to stand in this posture. I thought, *This is it! I am on my way. Now maybe I will learn to shoot lightning bolts out of my hands!* Nope, he just provided good instruction.

After showing me the specifics of standing in San Ti Shi, he told me to "just stand." Then he turned and walked away. He began teaching the other students. There was a group learning Chen Tai Chi Quan and a few students learning Ba Gua Quan. The group that was learning Tai Chi Quan were organized in rows and followed Sifu through the moves of the form. They were moving in unison and looked like a wave on the plaza. The people learning Ba Gua Quan were walking the circle. I had heard of the practice of walking the circle and it was intriguing to see it. I wanted to know more about it, but first I wanted to make sure I was learning all I could about Xing Yi Quan.

After a while I began to wonder if Sifu had forgotten about me. The lesson was about an hour, and I had been standing there for some time. I was pleased when Sifu did eventually come back, and he did a brief walk around me, made a few corrections to my hands and head, and then said, "Okay, keep it up." Then he left me to stand some more.

It was not a particularly hot day, but after a little while I could feel the sweat starting to run down my back. Several drops of sweat were cruising as slow and determined as snails to my waist, where they terminated in my clothes. My legs were feeling a weird mix of fatigue and energy circulation (at least that was how it felt). Sifu looked over to me and said, "Okay, change sides." He then went back to the other students and continued teaching Tai Chi Quan and Ba Gua Quan. I wondered how he could keep it all straight. It was like having plates in the air and he was able to keep us all spinning with ease. I was amazed at what he knew and how good a teacher he was. He never got upset. Even when people asked very pointed questions that I thought were a little brusque, he never got angry or agitated. He was very even, and I really liked that.

Sifu gave everyone their homework for the week, and came to me last. "Okay, looks good. Practice the standing this week, and I will give you something else next week." I then asked, "How long do I stand?" He was packing his bag to leave. He responded without missing a beat, "As long as you can." I began to think that I needed a better guideline. I told him that I was really busy, since I had recently become a new father and some days I can only manage a few minutes. He said, "Okay, stand for a few minutes." That sounded really logical but didn't give me the specific time I was looking for, so I told him some days I may only have a minute or two. He said, "Okay, then stand for a minute or two." All the while he was packing his bag and saying his pleasantries to students as they left. Now I was really puzzled. "Will that be enough?" I asked. He said, "Just be sure to do it every day. As long as you do it every day, you will build your foundation." I didn't realize then what a profound concept that would be in my life. Do a little, but do it every day.

This idea of a little at a time, but on a consistent basis, was not new to me, and yet I had not thought of applying it to all of the other areas of my life. I had been a musician and all of my best teachers had told me the same thing. It is not how long you do something, but how often. This is a really powerful concept to understand and adopt. The problem that most people have with it is that they think that a few minutes missed won't matter, but it does. The idea of making it up later doesn't really work. I hope that you incorporate this idea into other areas of your life as well, and you will find that things are more manageable and you will make progress.

Every week I would go to see Sifu and get my lesson. He taught me the forms, theory of generating power, and I was pleased to get to know him personally as well. He could answer any question and seemed to have a limitless supply of energy. He showed me the San Ti Shi and then the Five Element Form (which you'll learn from this book). Later I learned many forms that were not as well known. I told him I was very interested in the standing postures, and he showed me all he knew. I will always be grateful to Sifu Johnny Jang for being so free with his knowledge. I try to teach the same way.

I really enjoyed studying with Sifu Jang, and to this day he is one of my favorite teachers. He showed me the entire Xing Yi Quan system over a period of about three years, and eventually, he certified me as an instructor and presented me with a beautiful certificate which is hanging on my wall.

In addition to the Xing Yi Quan we would sometimes work on other styles. I told him that I was interested in all forms of standing, and he showed me all the Xing Yi Quan standing forms and many Yi Quan forms as well. I was curious and asked about Yi Quan, and he explained that it was similar to Xing Yi Quan but with even less material. Yi Quan is a great art, and Sifu related the main points to me, but I didn't want to get sidetracked, so I stayed with Xing Yi Quan.

My time was short as I was moving to Atlanta, so I would not be able to study with Sifu any longer. I let him know about my impending move and that I was sorry that I wouldn't be able to see him anymore. He was a great teacher, and we stayed in touch for a while, but my life became more focused on what I was doing with my new job and less with martial arts, so as happens with most of us, even with the best intentions, we drifted apart.

When I got to Atlanta and walked into our new house, I scouted it for a special location. I found a room that was away from the main living area. I declared to my wife, "I will do my standing in here." She just said, "Okay." I don't think she realized that I was telling *myself* as much as her that I wanted to continue my standing practice and develop my internal energy further.

I have continued studying and also practicing the rest of my Xing Yi Quan material. My favorite material to teach is the Qigong and Xing Yi Quan that I learned, and I love to see how people have improved their health and their lives. I hope you will find the same benefit.

How to use this book

Although the book is divided into postures for health and martial arts, these should not be thought of as mutually exclusive. They are simply divided into health and martial arts because that is how they are most often taught, and that is how I learned them. By using the postures from both categories you will enhance both your health and martial arts together. Martial arts skill and power will be enhanced by the health postures, and your health will benefit from the martial postures. Vigorous health enhances everything, of course, including your martial arts. So while there are specific postures for health and martial arts, they provide benefit for both areas, and you will obtain the most overall benefit when you practice them all.

There are many ways to do the postures that are in this book, and if you get instruction from another teacher, they may show you something slightly different. That is normal. You, as the student, just need to know that is not unusual and there are acceptable variations of most postures. You should always show respect to the teacher from whom you are learning, though, and do what they instruct. If you decide that you don't want to learn from them anymore, or find their differences too much, you should find a new instructor. I don't think it is ever acceptable to correct a teacher or give your opinion on what they are teaching. You should either study with them or move on.

I have included other subjects, such as partner participation and visualization exercises, that you may want to incorporate into your training. These subjects may be new to you, even if you have been studying standing Qigong, but I have found them extremely beneficial when teaching and practicing, and I encourage you to give them a try.

The focus of all instruction is to provide enough information so that you can begin standing correctly as soon as possible. I encourage you to read all of the sections, even if they may seem not to apply, as sometimes a piece of valuable information may jump out at you from an unlikely place.

PART I

HEALTH POSTURES

1

DIAPHRAGMATIC BREATHING

The breath is the best place to start. Practitioners of various arts and philosophies are often told to breathe from their diaphragm without ever being shown how to do it. I believe proper diaphragmatic breathing is the most powerful thing that you can do for your health, so I hope you take the time to do the exercises and incorporate diaphragmatic breathing into your practice and your life. You will notice a tremendous positive difference immediately.

Diaphragmatic breathing, also called abdominal breathing, is a form of breathing where the breath is done with expansion and contraction of the diaphragm. It is used in many disciplines including yoga, martial arts, and professional singing, as it is the best method to get the most oxygen into your body. Most people breathe shallowly and the breath is concentrated in their chest, but this method does not provide enough oxygen for the best results. Chest breathing is too shallow to provide enough air for deep breathing.

I first came across diaphragmatic breathing many years ago when I was learning to sing professionally. I was not able to project the way I needed to, and so my friend, who taught professionally, said that she could help me and showed me how. She told me that I would be louder, more in control, and I wouldn't get the sore throat or hoarse voice I had been getting from performing. I was skeptical but tried it out anyway, figuring that it couldn't really hurt. I thought it might be some kind of hocus pocus, but

I was pleasantly surprised. I could feel a real difference in the amount of air I was inhaling after learning to breathe properly, but I wondered how it would work for performing. Would it enable me to perform better?

We had a performance and I could absolutely feel the difference. I felt like I was projecting really well, and yet I was not out of breath like I had been. I was much more in control. At the end of the night, I felt good and didn't have the raspy, hoarse voice that I'd had before. I was definitely sold on the idea of diaphragmatic breathing for singing.

I was studying martial arts at the same time that I was playing music, and I had been told routinely to breathe from my diaphragm. My teacher would point to my abdomen to show me where to breathe, but not how to do it. I think most well-meaning people don't realize that without proper instruction, such as provided in this book, it is very difficult to do, if not impossible. The amount of oxygen was very noticeable and my body felt good and full of energy. I wasn't able to make the connection before, but now I could. When I practiced martial arts I found that I didn't get winded as quickly. It was a great feeling.

Most of us have not given much thought to how we breathe, so when following the instructions provided in this book the most important thing to do is to shift your awareness and really focus on what you are doing. Diaphragmatic breathing will feel different, but eventually this will feel natural and you will breathe this way all the time.

The simple exercise that follows is the best and quickest method to attain the skill of breathing diaphragmatically, and is the same one I learned. Follow the instructions carefully and take note that this breathing method will greatly enhance all parts of your life as well.

Diaphragmatic breathing process

1. Lie down on your back and relax. (A floor will work better than a bed.)

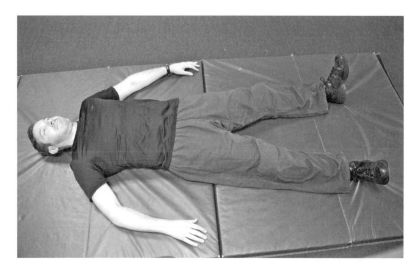

2. Put an object of some weight, such as a phone book or other small but somewhat weighty object, on your abdomen. Place the object so its middle is below your navel.

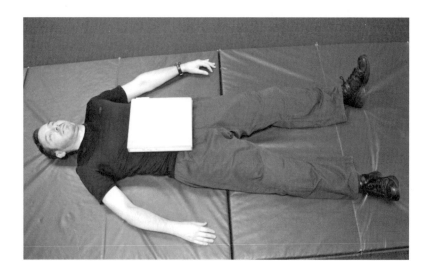

3. Breathe in deeply and push the object up as the air is entering your abdomen. Focus on raising the object with your diaphragm and expand/extend your abdomen. Make sure your chest and shoulders do not rise. Isolate the diaphragm area. (You may want to have a friend as a spotter to help.)

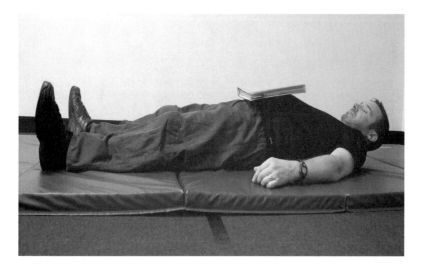

4. As you exhale watch the object float back down on your abdomen. Think of your empty abdomen as allowing the object to sink down low.

5. Follow steps 3 and 4 at least ten times, and each time try to inhale and exhale deeper.

6. You can use numbers if it is easier to keep track of the breaths. For the first breath, breathe in for a count of five and exhale for a count of five, then the next one can be six, and so forth.

7. If you have a spotter, watch that your chest and/or upper body is not moving or use a mirror. All of your concentration should be on the diaphragm and breath.

8. Once you have completed the repetitions, get up very slowly. Dizziness is common as you have been taking in more air than usual. First sit up carefully, and then take a moment before standing.

Now that you have learned this powerful new breathing method, you can try it in an exercise so that you can experience the difference. Incidentally, I mentioned that this method is taught to singers, but it is useful to anyone who needs to project their voice. When you take a deep breath, and then speak, you will notice that your voice has much more power. In martial arts this breathing enhances the "kiai" or martial arts yell that you hear the person perform when they are executing a technique. It helps to provide focus and power.

Breathing exercises

The exercises that follow are a great way to practice diaphragmatic breathing. You can also use them as a de-stressing exercise. The slow, deep breathing is very relaxing and calming. You may want to use them when you just "need a moment." For example, have you ever hit "reply to all" on an email, and you only meant to reply to one person? Maybe there was something in the email you wish you could take back, but now it is too late. You then feel that hot wave of panic and anxiety roll over your body. Knots form in your stomach and you realize that you have stopped breathing all together. These exercises are good to do in situations such as this.

You can try to recall that email, but also try this exercise while you wait. Breathe deeper each time, and eventually you should be able to calm down. It won't fix that email issue, of course, but you will be in a much better state of mind to deal with any issues that may arise from it.

Exercise 1

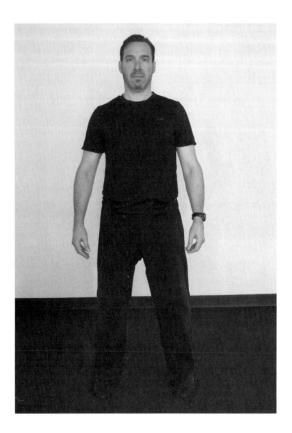

1. Stand in the natural posture as shown, with your feet the width of your shoulders. (You can also do this exercise seated, but you will likely find that it works best when standing.)

2. Place your hands over your abdomen (dan tien), just below your navel. You can close your eyes or allow them to remain open.

3. Breathe in and feel your hands being pushed away by your abdomen as it fills with air. Likewise, feel your hands fall as you exhale. Be sure not to press on your body with your hands, but rather let them lightly press against your

body just enough so you can feel your breath. (The hands are merely a way for you to gauge your breath, so they should not be exerting any effort or pressure.)

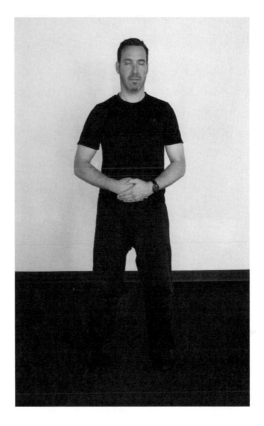

4. As you breathe you can count from one to five for the inhale, and five to one for the exhale. Raise the number gradually until you reach your limit. The goal is to have long, slender breaths, not to count to high numbers, so use the counting method only as a way to keep track of your breathing. If it becomes a distraction or fixation, stop using the counting method.

5. Do this exercise for about ten breaths, or as needed.

Exercise 2

Now you can also try the same posture, but let your hands hang by your sides.

1. Imagine that each breath brings you more energy and feel that the palms of your hands are warm.

2. Feel that your arms are charged with energy and gently bow out from your sides. Focus on your breath and feel your diaphragm expand and contract, but with no effort. You are merely aware of it working.

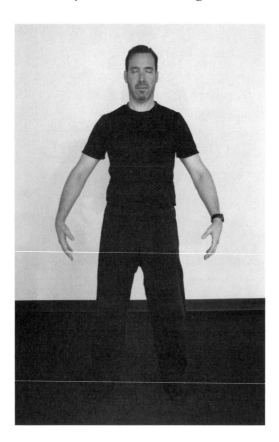

3. Gradually, focus on the breath only and nothing physical; just breathe.

Exercise 3

The following exercise is useful for helping you feel your body and breath together with very easy movements. This is a great exercise to start your day when you wake up, or to cleanse yourself of negative feelings and emotions. It can also be used to start or end your standing practice. Use it how it suits you best.

1. Stand in the Horse stance (see Chapter 3) with your arms by your sides for a few moments.

2. Inhale deeply and imagine your arms are floating up with the force and energy of your breath. Let your arms rise with your palms facing up.

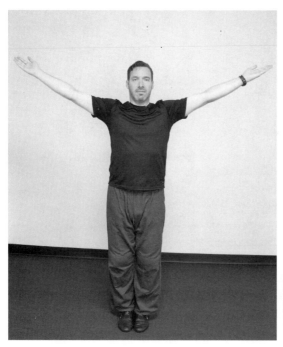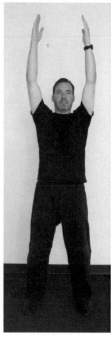

3. As your arms reach over your head in a large circle, let your palms face down. This should be done on the exhale of your breath.

4. Let the hands stay palms down as they pass in front of the center of your body. They should feel as though they are pushing out the breath as you exhale.

5. Once your hands reach the bottom (about waist level), let them float up with the inhale again.

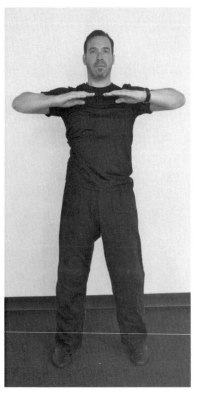
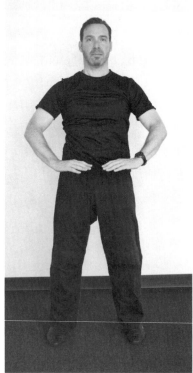

This whole exercise should look as though you are making a big circle with your arms. It is important to feel that your arms are light and that your breath is in fact making the arms rise over your head. Equally important is to feel that your exhale is pushing out the bad air as accompanied by your hands pushing down.

You can imagine taking in a breath with a great deal of energy, and when exhaling, releasing all bad energy or negativity as if cleansing your mind and body. One extremely important point is to match your motion to your breath and not your breath to your motion. You don't want to inhale because your arms are rising. Your arms are rising because you are inhaling. Always keep the breath as the most important part of all exercises and training (and the rest of your day, for that matter).

Now that you are able to breathe with the diaphragmatic method, you have completed the most important step. Always remember that nothing is more important than the breath, and it should always be a part of your practice of which you remain aware. Breathing is the most important focus in everything that you do. Breath is life. Apply this concept to other areas of your life and you will likely notice a pleasurable difference. Taking a few breaths before an important meeting or an undertaking that makes you nervous is underutilized but incredibly helpful.

2

PREPARATION FOR
HEALTH POSTURES

Now that you have learned diaphragmatic breathing, you will be able to really feel the difference in your standing Qigong practice. Because I feel that the breath is the most important thing, I devoted an entire chapter to it. As a teacher and student of standing Qigong and martial arts, I know that there are often other topics that come up regarding your study as well.

To some people, some of the topics may be seemingly unrelated until you read them in context. As a teacher I have addressed many topics, but I have included only the most commonly covered topics in this chapter. They are presented to you in a way that you can get the most out of the book. This chapter demonstrates how I teach standing Qigong, and I hope it makes your practice more enjoyable.

Visualization

One of the most powerful tools that we have is visualization. It is such a powerful technique that it is used in professions of all kinds including sports and healing therapies. The picture you create in your mind is often as powerful as, or even more powerful than, what you see in front of you.

Most of the directions in this book require you to visualize. In some cases you are asked to visualize parts of your body or energy working a particular way. Some things are known and easy to do. Some things are imagined and require more thought and attention.

The one certainty with visualization is that it works very well in many ways. While you are using the standing postures you use visualization to get your body into alignment and to tell the various parts of your body what to do or how to feel. This is a very instructive way to think into the posture. I feel visualization is so important that I have included a section with a few visualization exercises so that you can experiment with the method (see Chapter 6).

I want to share one of the most powerful moments I ever had with standing Qigong and also with visualization. I was using it to treat my anxiety. I was becoming a real anxious person for no apparent reason. I felt that I needed to do something. I went to my friend who had introduced me to standing Qigong, and told him about my dilemma. He asked if I was still doing the standing, and I said I was. He asked if it helped, and I said that I still felt anxious for some reason. He asked me when I didn't feel anxious. I told him when I practiced martial arts I felt good and had no anxiety. He then told me to visualize myself doing martial arts when I was standing. I wasn't sure what he meant. "Do you mean picture myself doing techniques and things?" I asked. He said, "Yes."

His theory was that if I was visualizing myself doing something that I felt strong and confident doing, that it should make me actually feel that way and relieve the anxiety. I tried it that day and didn't notice anything, but I also felt I probably hadn't given it as good a try as I could. I waited until the next day and then tried again. Once I was standing in the posture, I started to see myself doing the techniques and things that I liked to do. I was visualizing in slow motion, and I don't know if it mattered, but that is what I did.

I became lost in the images. Slowly and effortlessly I could see myself performing everything in amazing detail. All the while I felt really good. I felt like I was really there, doing it at that moment. In the middle of an amazing feat of skill my timer went off, and I was back to the present moment. I felt really good. I used this method consistently until I didn't feel that I needed to use it to treat anxiety any longer. After reading about Olympic athletes visualizing for performance, I began using the same method to improve my martial arts skills.

My standing practice was taken to the next level as I incorporated visualization. If you are already a visualization practitioner, you are ahead of the game. If you have never practiced visualization, it is very powerful and will yield results if you try it.

Exercise

Limbering up your body in any way you want is good preparation. I suggest basic stretching as illustrated in the introduction to the health postures (see Chapter 3). Keep in mind that these are merely suggestions, and if you would like to use other exercises that serve the same purpose, then you should use what you prefer.

The most important thing is that you move your body. Through standing Qigong your body is gaining energy and you are using muscles, but in a different way. As you are standing on your legs, be sure to rotate your ankles and hips, but also your arms, neck, and all the other parts of your body.

Basic stretching is important whether you practice standing Qigong or not. With disuse the muscles atrophy and you lose mobility. The best rule to remember for your body and how to treat it is, "What have you done for me lately?" It doesn't matter if in your youth you were active, although that is good. Inactivity will only harm your body. You should not use age as an excuse either. By starting small and building strength through standing,

I hope you will also learn the Five Element Form (see Chapter 5), as that is a great place to start incorporating movement into your practice.

I teach many people who are over the age of 80 and mobility is an issue. Some things are not preventable, but many physical issues can be prevented with even the most modest physical activity. If this book is part of your new focus on self-improvement and physical fitness, I applaud you. Start now, and be happy with the fact that you have done what so many have not and will not: embarked on a new beginning.

The body works best when moved every day. The joints are especially important. Rotate your arms at the shoulder and your legs at the hips slowly through their full range of motion daily and you will likely keep them free from injury and atrophy. It is easy to do, but as the great motivational speaker Jim Rohn used to say, "It's also easy not to do." Therein lies the difference between a great deal of success and failure. While watching TV you can drop and do pushups until the show comes back on, or you can stand in the Tiger posture, or you can stay on your bottom while that infernal commercial plays on, and watch as if strapped to the chair. We all have a choice.

I used to run at a lakeside park by my house for a while, and I was always fascinated by this one woman who used to come and practice her martial arts. I would make my circuit by where she would practice, so within a lap I would see her park and unpack her martial arts weapons. She would unpack a staff from a long case, as well as a spear. Then she would pull out some short-range weapons. There may have been more, but I saw a straight sword and a broad sword, as well as a whip chain. She would start with the shorter-range weapons and practice her sets of those before moving to the long weapons. It looked like she had sets from a variety of arts. As I would run I could see her practicing faintly from across the lake. She would go directly from one weapon to the next. I noticed that she would occasionally focus on a particular sequence of movements and then do the set all together. I had quite a few laps to complete, so I was disappointed when she left. I enjoyed watching her practice. She practiced for about 20–30 minutes, although sometimes more and sometimes less. She was consistent, though. She did a little often rather than a lot all at once.

The lesson learned from watching the woman at the park is that by choosing something where you are constantly striving for improvement, it is intellectually interesting and also satisfying. By practicing the sets she was putting her body through a complete range of motion and using every part of it. Because it did not take very long, she could fit it into her schedule. All of these items are worthy of note, and you should think about them as you put an exercise routine into practice.

Energy

The concept of energy in any other context than fuel for your car or electricity for your home is often scoffed at by Western civilization. I can illustrate what I mean with a short anecdote. I once commented to some friends that someone seemed to have a real negative energy, and my friends laughed out loud. "What are you, some kind of hippie?" I was a little surprised. I asked them what they meant. They told me that energy is something that hippies or New Age people talk about. They were not referring to these types of people in a positive way; these were meant to be derogative terms. I was caught off guard because it seemed that energy should not be that controversial. They then commented that since I was interested in that "Eastern stuff," they thought it made sense. I was a little stunned by their reaction, but I realized that in the West, we don't really think too much about our bodies, or how they work. Anything outside the mechanics and nuts and bolts of the body often seems to be deemed as weird by most people not introduced to Qigong or martial arts.

Let me start by saying that Qigong means energy work, and that there are many ways of expressing what the energy of the body is called. You can call it chi (now often called qi), ki, internal energy, prana, bioelectric energy, power of intention, and more terms that I haven't learned yet. They are all the same thing. Internal energy is real energy, although some of the claims of such energy can put people off, and I understand why. Some of the stories of abilities related to chi are more than a little far-fetched. My friend and I embarked on an odyssey into all esoteric martial arts to see what we could find, and we did come across some good things and some bad things. We met some incredible learned teachers who imparted great wisdom to us, and some complete charlatans who supplied us with a chuckle or two by claiming to possess abilities that I have only seen in movies with great special effects.

I once read that a well-known martial arts expert didn't believe in qi. I realized that what he meant was that he didn't believe some of the extraordinary claims people have made about qi. As I have stated, I agree; however, there is such a thing as energy and we all possess it. The energy of the body is real. I had to enlighten my friends who were dubious about the concept of energy—what did they think a defibrillator was for? What is an electrical synapse in the body? The body is full of energy. The body conducts electricity. Energy is all around us. When you focus your mind with intention you can feel the difference. You can feel real tangible results.

Energy is often easily or most easily felt and obvious when you practice Qigong with others. When you practice on your own, you are working solely with *your* energy, but when you work with others, your energy joins with the other participants, and you get more powerful energy. As with most things, when you have people with similar goals and efforts, you get more results. I would caution people only to make sure that they practice with someone they genuinely like or that they feel good being around.

When I conduct my classes, and we have many students, you can really feel the energy level. First-time students often volunteer that they really felt "something" when they were standing. I have one student who has a chronic illness that causes fatigue, and she said that she can immediately feel the difference when she comes to the class. She always feels a great deal better. I am cautious about suggesting someone may feel something so as to avoid feelings being attributed to mere suggestion. I prefer to let the student volunteer what they are feeling if anything at all.

When discussing energy and how it interacts with yourself and others, you don't have to think just about practicing Qigong or martial arts. It can be as simple as sharing a meal with someone. If you eat with someone you enjoy spending time with, you will find the meal more satisfying than eating alone. Growing up I remember eating meals that probably violated most of the ways people think about nutrition for children, but they still enabled me to grow into a healthy person. My mother cooked our meals, and when a loved one like a mother or father prepares food for their family, they are putting that extra ingredient of themselves into the food. They are putting in their energy. I don't want to digress into a diatribe of contemporary American society, but perhaps the loss of the home-cooked meal is why we have such nutritional and dietary problems today.

I hope you will not think of energy, be it called chi, qi, or anything else, as so mystical as to be considered esoteric. As you get in tune with your body, you will feel the effects of energy and the benefits as well.

Religion

Qigong and martial arts have origins in the East and have roots in various forms of Eastern religions such as Taoism and Buddhism. I respect all religions, but when I teach, I prefer to leave out religion all together and focus on the actual postures and forms themselves, and how they can provide the most benefit. Religion need not be a part of martial arts or Qigong, and I don't teach any religious ideas when I instruct. When it comes to this subject, people can make their own choice. For example, when students come to learn from me they almost always ask if I am going to be talking about Eastern religion, chanting, and so forth. They often point out that they follow a particular religion, and that they have put off learning Qigong or martial arts because they feared having to deal with a particular opposing religion. They are always relieved when I tell them that what they are learning is a non-religious program of postures for health and martial arts.

Anyone can learn and benefit from the postures, and it is my sincere hope that many people will try them out and make them a regular practice as part of their exercise, regardless of any philosophy.

Music

I have heard much about the use of music. I have heard you shouldn't have any. I have heard you should have music, but only a certain kind. Music is good. Music is bad. To all of this I say, 'Rubbish!' Do what you want. There is no right or wrong if it is pleasurable to you and helps you to achieve your goal.

I personally use Gregorian chant and the music of Hildegard low in the background when I teach my classes, as well as other forms of classical music. I was once a musician and I still enjoy music, so I won't banish it from my practice just because someone doesn't approve. Also I have found that music can cushion the extraneous sounds if you are in a noisy place. My school is next to a location that has many events, and the walls are quite thin. Having some music to cover up the other sounds makes them less intrusive.

A student once asked me if I had special music, as he had seen a Tai Chi Quan music CD. I told him I didn't have special music, and he was surprised. He asked me what kind of music he should use. I asked him if he likes having music while he stands, and he said, "No." I said, "Then don't have music." He asked, "But don't I have to?" I was a bit surprised, but knowing that most of us want to be good rule followers, we sometimes forget that we have choices, and often you should simply do what you want. If you enjoy a particular type of music, you should use it, but if you don't want music, don't have any.

There is also the music of nature. It sounds clichéd, but I think getting outside once in a while is a good idea. Standing by a river or stream, hearing the birds and other natural sounds, is a nice diversion from all of the artificial sounds that surround us daily. If you can't go outside to nature, try a nature CD playing low while you stand. In some cases you just need to open a window or door and let the outside in.

Distractions

When my son was a child, the only time I could practice standing was when he was watching a children's show on TV. I would practice my standing behind the couch and try to tune out the TV, which was filled with children's music, and only focus on him and myself. I found this to be a very useful exercise and challenging as well. It is extremely difficult to tune things out, but as I said, it was a useful exercise. If I were to have waited for a time when there were no distractions, I probably never would have done anything at all.

It is true, and certainly preferable, that a quiet place is best, but that is not always possible. Rather than let our circumstances control us, we can control our circumstances by simply adapting to the situation at hand. If you find that the only time and place to stand is a noisy back room of a warehouse in your building, then use it. Try your best to concentrate on what you are doing, without thinking about what else is happening around you. The key to tuning things out is to think about what you are doing to the exclusion of everything else.

Go through the inventory of items in your head of how to hold the posture, and use your visualizations if possible. Feel your body and focus on your breath. Before you know it, you are in your own world and enjoying your self-created island of peace.

Attitude

Your attitude is probably the most important aspect of your practice. Why do you want to practice standing? What do you want to accomplish? These are your goals. They are yours alone. No matter how much instruction you receive from this book or a teacher, you should never lose sight of your goals with your practice.

You must not practice to satisfy anyone but yourself. Standing is meditative, so your focus will always be inward once the mechanics are obtained. This means that you will eventually come face to face with yourself, and hopefully you will find this meaningful, helpful, enlightening, and pleasant. For some people this may be the very first time doing an activity with inward reflection. This may be a truly new experience for you, and I hope you will continue, as we all need moments of inward focus.

Most people abandon a new activity rather quickly after it doesn't produce results quick enough. Those that stick with something new are the ones who succeed. If you purchased this book, you obviously have the interest, so I hope you will stay with it. One only has to speak to someone with a gym membership that is not being used to have a very good idea of the power of attitude.

I knew someone who had a gym membership and had gone a few times the first week with a great deal of enthusiasm. She was trying to lose weight, so she would weigh herself each day. The second or third week she was discouraged at not seeing the progress that she wanted to see. She eventually gave up. I was very sad to see this happen, because I don't think that she ever really gave it a chance. I have always thought that while it takes time to gain the weight, it takes at least as long to lose it. By setting unrealistic expectations with an improper attitude we set ourselves up for failure.

I have noticed as a student and teacher that the ones who stick to something tend to approach it gradually. I think that this is the best way to do most things. I don't mean to put a damper on anyone's enthusiasm; I just want to caution against too much too soon. Be in it for the long haul, and always keep a long-term vision of your goals. When you slowly add a minute or two per week to your overall standing, in a very short amount of time, you will be standing for longer than you had probably imagined. This method will serve you well in all parts of your life, so I hope you will try it.

Food and bodily functions

I don't recommend standing after eating, or if you are particularly weak from illness. Standing is best practiced when you are neither full nor hungry, as both can be distractions. Treat standing like a long trip in the car, and use the restroom before you get started. Also, like with a long trip, don't eat a big meal or drink a great deal right before. Don't drink alcohol before or immediately after standing.

You don't have to start on a diet to start standing, but you may want to consider healthier food choices. If you eat two donuts every morning, maybe one morning you should eat one donut and substitute an apple for the second one. I love what is commonly called comfort foods, such as meatloaf, fried eggs, burgers, fries, and all the rest, but I know that I can't eat it every day without there being some serious repercussions to my health. Especially as we get older we need to consider alternatives. I am a big believer in moderation, so I am not suggesting the elimination of the things you really love, but simply alternating with other things once in a while.

Most of us learn our eating habits as children, and they don't change much as we get older. If this is the case with you, and you haven't changed anything since you were young, consider healthier alternatives sometimes. Our relationship to food is at least as important as the form of exercise we choose.

We need to use common sense with food. If you are over 40 and you eat 1000 calories and only burn 500, there is some pretty simple math to consider, and all of the justification in the world won't change the facts.

Food is fuel and energy. It does matter what you put in your body. In addition to a healthy diet, you may want to consider taking vitamins. I used to feel really run down until I started taking vitamins. Lately, I know that taking any supplements has become controversial, but as with everything, we should consider moderation. The place where I usually get myself into trouble is the extremes. The moderate path in most things has been maligned, but I have found that it is best for me and seems easiest to govern.

One thing that I do that I didn't realize was different is that I never eat food hot or cold. I eat just about everything room temperature. This has been to the complete frustration of most of my friends and family who are food connoisseurs. (I am definitely not a "foodie" as they are called.) I like to eat without burning my mouth or chilling my brain and teeth into a deep freeze, so I usually wait for a bit before eating or drinking anything until it is about room temperature. You may want to try it, as it seems easier on the digestion. It also requires a bit of patience, and we sometimes need to practice that as well.

Location

A place that has an open feel and fresh, cool air is best, but don't feel limited by this suggestion. What is best is not always available, so try to find the best place you can. When you begin, a place that can be used consistently is best. You want to avoid distraction when getting started, so keep that in mind. In time, you can test your "tuning out skills," but that will be difficult when first starting.

When you choose a location you should also take into account the availability of the location. Remember, consistency is the key. If you choose an outside location, make sure that it is available all year long. If you live in a location with extreme weather changes, decide to either incorporate them into your practice or choose another location. If you have a location that is good only for a few days a year, choose somewhere else. Don't set yourself up for failure.

Outside locations are good to experiment with, though, and I do recommend trying to use them when weather permits. I used to hike up a very large hill by my house and do my standing practice at the top. The air is clean, and the only noises are natural. You can hear the wind blow by your ears and the rustling of the leaves and bushes. The sun on your face, the wind blowing against your skin, and the natural sounds of birds are all a very pleasant diversion from our indoor lives.

Indoors can be challenging as well, but often the challenges are more easily overcome. There was a time when I couldn't practice standing at home, so I found an open conference room in my building at work and used it early in the morning. I used to put a sign out that said "Meeting in Progress" to avoid interruption. Keep this in mind when choosing your location, that home may not be the best place, and that you can stand anywhere.

If you are going to use a place in your home, and you want to avoid distraction, you may need to tell family members to leave you alone for a while so that you can practice. Don't be self-conscious about doing this. Everybody has a right to do the things that they need to do to accomplish their goals. Having a few moments to yourself is not selfish. It is good for you and those around you.

Disconnect from everything. Turn off that phone and put it somewhere else. If this is difficult for you, I suggest you do it more often whether practicing standing or not. To realize how much time we all spend on meaningless endeavors, perform an experiment: keep track of what you actually do with your phone and how meaningful (as in important) those actions are. You will probably find, as most people do, that we all spend a great deal of time on things that are neither important, meaningful, nor time-sensitive, yet we have all been conditioned to think that they are. This may be the subject of another book, but until then, try this experiment.

Time

When are you going to start? What time are you going to do it? The time you choose is as important as the location. You should try to choose a time that you can stick to, and be honest about it. If you are usually pretty groggy in the morning and you can barely drag yourself out of bed, don't choose the morning to do your standing practice. You will likely do it a few times and then abandon it. Instead, think about when you have a spare moment. Is there a small space of time that you can use where no one will intrude? Is there a time of day when the kids are at their friend's house? Be creative and honest about when you will be able to do it, and then stick to it.

You can choose night, morning, or the middle of the day—it makes no difference—just choose a time that you will be able to keep consistently, and then keep to it. If you decide to do your practice at work, resist the urge to miss it because there is a crisis. There will always be a crisis. There will always seemingly be something more important, but in reality, very few things are as important as we think they are. Stick to your time and, like your location, make it sacred. For those few minutes focus on your goal of internal development.

Duration

How long should you hold each posture? That is up to you to decide. Start with a minute and work up from there. However, if you have a difficult time holding the posture for a minute, then do what you can. This is where you need to be honest with yourself as well. Don't give up easily, but don't coerce yourself when you are not ready. It is a delicate balancing act of looking into yourself and being honest.

For some of us this is the most difficult part of studying anything. When things are new they are usually difficult, and our bodies and minds sometimes start working on us a bit. The good thing is that as soon as you push through and make a commitment to your new endeavor, and it becomes your new habit, you will start to feel the opposite.

Use the mental directives and techniques that you will learn in this book to help you. Remember that you are not competing with anyone and there is no real winner or loser unless you start thinking in this fashion. Consistent practice and incremental increases in the duration of your practice will provide you with success, as it does with most things.

Clothes

"What do I wear?" That is a very common question regarding Qigong practice. Wear what is comfortable. I can honestly say I have no fashion sense—I look about the same all the time— nor do I concern myself with the latest martial arts fashions. My thoughts on clothes are that they should be comfortable and functional and that is all. You don't need special shoes, pants, or shirts.

I used to work next door to a store that sold yoga fashions, and I couldn't believe what they had in there. There were so many different kinds of pants, shirts, and shoes that I was overwhelmed. (I studied yoga with a teacher and we just wore sweats!) I am sure some of it is functional, but most of it looked like it was meant to impress fellow students. I wondered how many people don't practice yoga because they don't have the latest fashion, or because they feel self-conscious wearing some of the clothes. It is not just with yoga, though. I have seen martial arts studios with elaborate uniforms, and some studios that require different-colored uniforms for different ranks or purposes. Everyone is entitled to do what they want, and if it works for them, great, but I really think the focus should be on the activity. I know that similar dress promotes more of a feeling of cohesion and unity in a group of people, but we should not forget that martial arts, and most other related activities, are about individual achievement.

I once had a student tell me that they showed up for class but that they went home because they forgot their uniform. I told them to never do that again. Always remember that *you* are the most important thing, not your uniform or clothes. I reminded him that he won't likely be wearing his uniform when he has to use his martial arts, so he shouldn't worry about forgetting it.

Sometimes we get caught up in what others are doing, or what we have been told, and forget the basics. What are the basics? Focus on what is most important. I used to run, and my wife would cringe when I left the house because I would wear some really old cut-off sweat pants with holes in them. The shirt was old with a controversial message, so I wore it inside out. The shoes also had holes, but they were really comfortable. I would go for my run looking a bit like Oliver Twist, but it never bothered me. I would see people with the latest running fashions, but I noticed I didn't see them that often. I am not passing judgment, but merely making an observation.

The old saying "the clothes make the man" was likely coined by a tailor, so don't worry about it. *You make yourself*, and nothing else does. I think back to the first time I practiced standing in that parking lot. People were driving by and probably looking, but we just focused on what we were doing. Why does anyone care what a stranger thinks? For that matter, why does anyone care what *anyone* thinks? Focus on yourself.

With all of that said, I suppose I would be remiss not to recommend *something*, though, so I suggest sweat-type pants and a t-shirt. Shoes just need to be comfortable, so running or walking shoes are fine. If you have good feet (for example, no fallen arches), you may want to try practicing standing barefoot. It is completely up to you. Whatever you do, don't put up barriers to starting with ideas like, "I don't have anything to wear!"

3

HEALTH POSTURES

The health postures included in this book are in no way to be considered the only ones. They are merely the ones I have been taught, and there are variations of them as well as different postures altogether. In the world of Qigong and martial arts there are often many ways to do one thing, and alternatives should be accepted as just that—alternatives—and not looked upon negatively.

All of the postures involve the idea of holding and interacting with a sphere, or ball. In the beginning it may be helpful to think of a regular ball that you have played with, and then eventually when using visualization we can include different directives and ways of thinking of the ball as a sphere of energy or hollow, and so forth.

Although these postures are probably best practiced as a set, don't think that you must always practice them all at the same time. You can also just practice one or two and they will provide you with great benefit. I am not a big believer in "legalistic" ways of practicing Qigong, and I don't want you to think of the guidelines as "unbreakable laws." They are simply guidelines and suggestions. Once you start practicing, feel free to experiment.

Although these postures are grouped and labeled as health postures, that does not limit their use. They benefit practitioners of martial arts as well. As these postures are a little easier to learn than the martial postures, martial arts practitioners may want to start here to build up some of the feelings and basics of standing Qigong before attempting the more demanding martial postures.

Horse stance

The Horse stance used in the health stances is not the same as the one often used in traditional martial arts. This stance is much shorter and a little taller. If you have ever seen the martial arts movies where the student is standing in a really low stance with tea cups on his thighs, and is instructed that he cannot spill any tea, that is a more extreme Horse stance. This stance should find your feet at just about shoulder width. I recommend using a mirror when checking the details of the stances as often a mirror will provide irrefutable evidence of what you are actually doing, and to ensure that your practice is productive, you need to see what you are doing *exactly*.

The easiest way to get your feet to the proper position is to follow the instructions provided below.

1. Start with your feet together (next to each other).

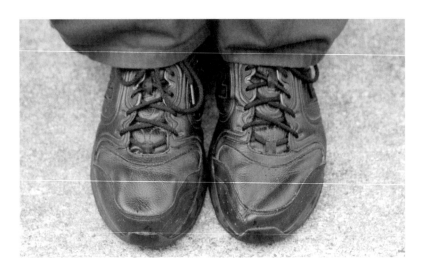

2. Push your heels out as far as possible while keeping your toes pointing at each other. Pivot on the ball of your foot.

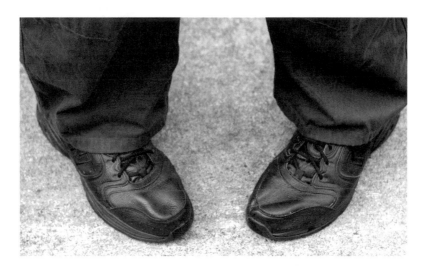

3. Straighten your toes so that your feet are separated and your toes are facing forward. The feet should be parallel and not pointing out away from each other.

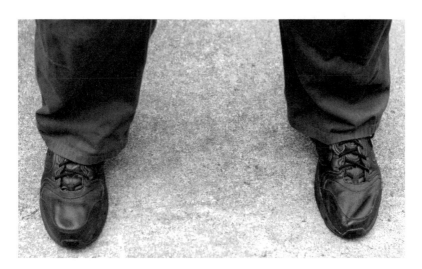

If this is new to you, you need to be extra diligent about the placement of the feet. An easy way to check your feet are in the right position is to place your hands straight in front of you with your fingers together, facing front, palms down. Look down at your feet and make your feet point straight like your hands.

This stance is used for all of the health postures, so re-read this section if necessary to ensure you have a good foundation for the stance. When the Horse stance is referred to in this book, this is what is being referenced.

This a powerful position for your body. You likely normally stand in a position that is similar to this, so with some modifications you will feel it as a natural part of your body.

Alignment

The alignment of your body physically and your mind mentally is integral to everything—not only in Qigong, but also in life. The standing postures can be seen as a metaphor for life. If you are still, aligned, and filled with the intention for whatever you wish to accomplish, you will be successful. However, the opposite is also true. If you are not mindful of your internal or external self, little or nothing positive is likely to materialize. When starting the physical alignment I find it is easier to start from the bottom and work your way up, so I start with the feet.

The feet should be placed first, then the hips, shoulders, and finally the head. In the health postures these parts of your body are all virtually the same; however, in the martial postures they are all quite different. When you get to that section (see Chapter 4), pay particular attention to how you get into the posture.

The main thing to keep in mind when thinking about your alignment is where your center of balance, or "center," is located. Always think of the feet and hips as the foundation of each posture and then build onto them. The shoulders will usually want to rise a bit, so you will need to think of dropping them.

Think about the head as floating up. Imagine a string pulling up the head from the back. Your head will rotate slightly up and your chin will move in a little. (You don't want a military-style chin tuck, though.) Use imagery to visualize a gradual rotation of your head in and up. Use a mirror or partner to check that it is correct. Once you know what it should feel like, try to remember the feeling.

All of the standing postures have your arms in various shapes, but one thing is constant throughout most of the postures, with some exceptions, and that is, that your hands are in the center of your body. Usually, they are in front of your chest area. This area is your power zone. This is where your hands are in the strongest position in relation to your body.

If you try this simple exercise, you will be able to feel the strength of having your hands in the proper position.

1. Bring your hands in front of your chest and press the palms together. Point the fingers away from you.

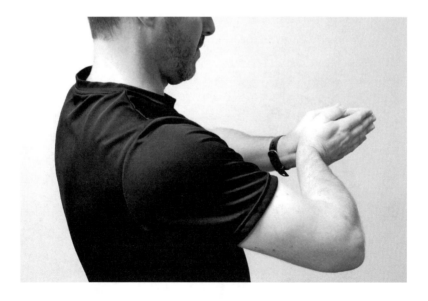

2. While pressing the palms together, push your hands away from you (extend your arms). You will notice it feels weak.

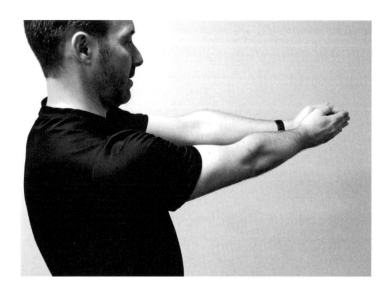

3. Draw back your hands toward your chest and stop when they feel strong. You will notice that you likely have stopped in front and rather close to your chest. That is your power zone for your hands.

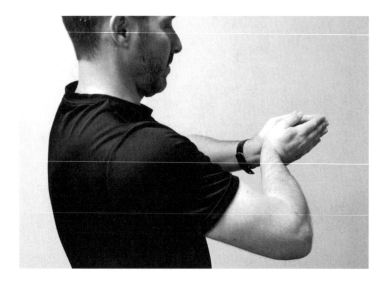

Your hands are strong in this position, because they are in alignment with your body. There are a few exceptions, but the best rule to follow is to keep your hands in front of you. Be sure that they are neither too low nor too high. Equally important is to make sure that they are not too close or too far either. The "Goldilocks Zone" that astrophysicists refer to when looking for planets like the Earth is a good rule of thumb for most things: Find the middle ground.

You should not feel stiff, but if this is the first time you have given your posture much thought, it will probably feel a little strange, and most students' first reaction is to monitor everything so closely that it becomes somewhat unnatural. I am a fan of the old school of just about everything and I still think walking with a book on your head is a great way to fix your posture. After you stand for a time, try it out. I think you will find it enjoyable, helpful, and challenging.

Aligning your mind with your body is essentially the purpose of standing Qigong. You are using mental directives and images to get into the posture. Unlike most Western exercise where the mind is completely disconnected, with standing Qigong and all other forms of Qigong we are integrating our mind. In fact, the most common reason people tell me that they don't go to the gym is because they are bored. With standing Qigong, once you are well versed and comfortable with your ability to hold the postures, you can start experimenting with using visualization techniques such as the ones described in this book.

Internal and external definitions

The terms *internal* and *external* can become murky, so I will define them as clearly as I can in the context of martial arts, Qigong, and my experience, and hopefully they will be easier to understand. Internal refers to the mental component of what you are doing, whereas external is more physical. This is an extremely broad way to describe these terms, but it is a good place to start.

Qigong of all types has an internal component, where you use your mind to do the exercise. Compare this idea to a jumping jack, which for the most part is completely physical. Now that I have used these two examples, though, I can think of many exceptions to both. Mixed martial arts are considered a very external form of martial arts, but some of the fighters actually have a very internal approach. Likewise, there are many practitioners of internal arts who focus so much on the particulars of what they are doing that they forget to feel, breathe, and use their mind, and so it becomes an empty dance.

The art I studied originally has both internal and external components, and would be hard to categorize as a purely external art, though it usually is. The three main internal arts—Xing Yi Quan, Ba Gua Quan, and Tai Chi Quan—are all known to be internal, and so they are, but often, when students get better acquainted with the arts, they are surprised by some of the physicality. Nothing really falls neatly in either camp, but rather most combine elements of both.

To Western minds, it has been my experience that people equate internal with easy and soft. These are two ideas that an art such as Xing Yi Quan can seemingly defy, so we often need to look deeper than the various labels and think more about what we are doing. The last and most obvious point to make is that one orientation is not better than the other, except in the context of what you are trying to achieve and what your goals are.

Intention and awareness

Often in the instructions for the various postures I mention shifting your intention or awareness to a specific area. For instance, while holding the postures you will be instructed to think about the area in front of you, below, behind, and so forth. You will not be actually moving in any direction but rather making subtle and imperceptible changes. The feeling is internal. A simple way to understand this concept is to have a partner gently push against your posture while you hold it. The first thing students often do is lean in the direction upon which they are focusing. Be aware and correct this so that there is no lean. In all of the postures you should remain straight up and down. The shift is completely internal.

You can have your partner gently push against your arms while you hold the postures, and feel that with no thought of stiffening to them, you are holding your arms in the proper position. A helpful way to think of your body, while testing your posture, is that it is filled with energy that is circulating through your body. Imagine energy is circulating through your arm and that is what holds it in position, and it will be almost immovable.

Preparatory exercises

Pivot the body

This is the first exercise and is the best for all-around purposes. It will help you feel your body, as well as loosen it up. Relaxation is the key. Let the motion relax the entire body. The most critical thing to remember is that the lower body is moving the upper body.

1. Stand in the Horse stance and imagine your head floating up. Think of a pole going through the center of your body and keeping everything in alignment.

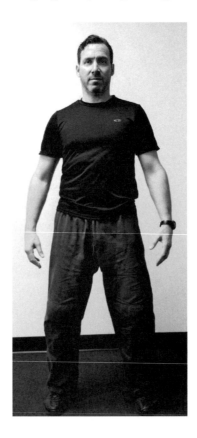

2. With your right foot, push so that your hip turns to the left and your arms gently slap at your sides. Then do the same with your left foot so that your hip turns to the right.

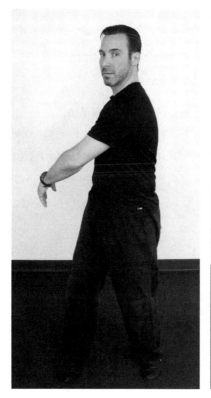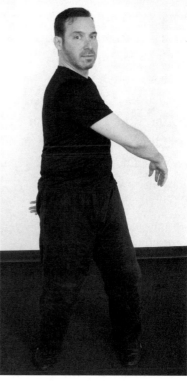

3. Gradually increase the speed so that you are gently turning by pushing with your feet, alternating left and right. Push from the edges of the feet. Keep your head looking straight ahead.

4. As you turn watch that your hips don't sway back and forth.

5. Check that your feet are always straight, and correct them if they are pointing in different directions.

6. I don't suggest any particular number of repetitions; merely do it for a few minutes.

This is an amazing exercise. It can help you feel alignment while using motion, as well as help you feel driving (pushing) with your legs. I use this exercise every day and I start every class with it. It is deceptively easy, so watch for the common mistakes of swaying or moving your arms instead of letting them be moved by your body.

The basis of this exercise is the foundation of all of the health postures, so it is a good one to do before practicing, even if you decide not to do any others. Be sure to spend some time with this exercise and check it with a partner or a mirror to make sure you have it down correctly.

Touch your toes

This is the old-school exercise of touching your toes, but with a new twist. Usually when this exercise is done, certainly when I learned it in my elementary school physical education class, people bend primarily at the waist, grit their teeth, and try stretching harshly. With some slight modification this can be a more productive exercise.

Still reach down for your toes, but think about rolling down your spine instead of merely bending at the waist. Start at your head and roll down. When you get to the limit, think of reaching with a relaxed stretch. Similarly think about rolling back up as well.

As you roll down be sure to exhale and reach for your toes. Relax. A few repetitions are enough. Each time try to reach a little farther. You should feel the stretch in the back of your legs and calves.

If you are familiar with the yoga posture "the plow," this is similar, although it is done standing. In the same way that you roll your body over in that posture, you roll your body down in this one.

Rotate your hips: part 1

Rotating your hips is a challenging exercise, so be sure to go slow and don't do too much too soon. The exercise is presented in two parts. As I have become older, I have found I use this exercise more, and it feels great. I have a student with a hip issue and this exercise really helps.

1. Take a really wide stance with your feet as far apart as possible. Keep your feet facing forward so that you are using the edges of your feet, the same as in the Horse stance.

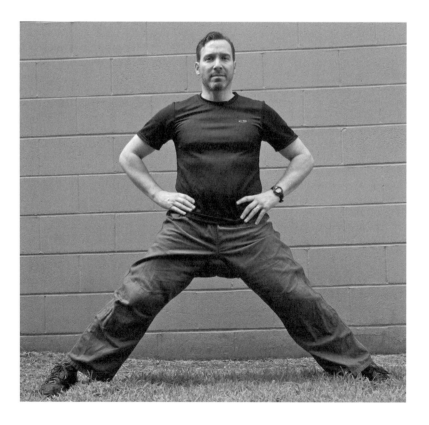

2. Gently push with your left foot and turn as far as possible to the right. Hold the position for a few breaths.

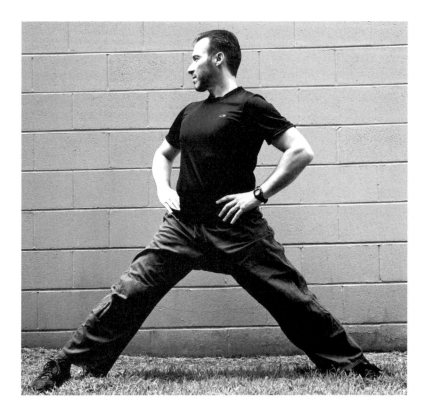

3. Now gently push with your right foot and turn to your left as far as possible. Again, hold the position for a few breaths.

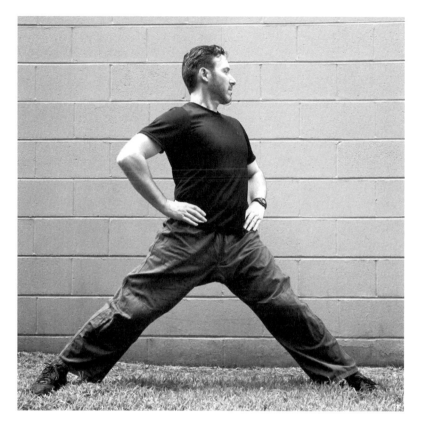

4. Do about three repetitions on each side.

Rotate your hips: part 2

1. As you exhale, keep your feet pushing to the edges. Relax your upper body.

2. Cross your arms.

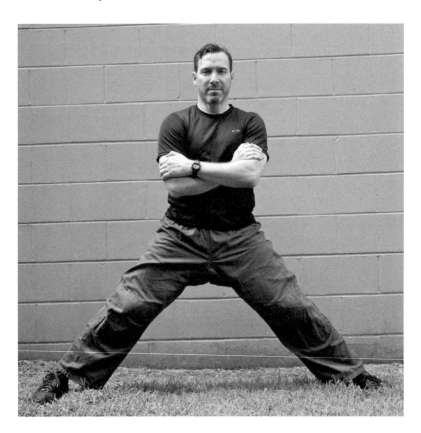

3. Roll your upper body down and rotate your hips down. Let your body hang upside down for a few breaths with your crossed arms hanging as well.

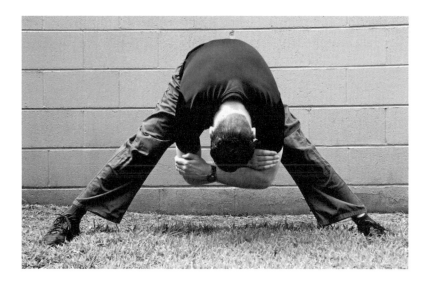

4. Use your legs and hips to roll your body back up again.

5. The whole exercise should be done slowly.

6. Do about three repetitions.

To get out of the wide stance, use your hands to "walk your body." Place your hands on the floor and take little steps away from your feet with your hands, as if walking forward. This will gently bring your body closer to the ground and you can then bring your legs together. Position your legs and hips underneath you and then stand up. This is a great exercise to do a few times a week.

Whether you do all or some of the exercises is up to you, but you should do some kind of preparatory exercise before standing in the postures. You may also want to use some of the exercises *after* standing as well. Always listen to your body, and do what you need. Start with my suggestions and then tailor them. The important thing is that you do some kind of preparatory exercise before standing in the postures.

Health postures

Holding the sphere

As I mentioned previously, this group of standing postures can be practiced together as a set or individually. The value of doing the entire set is great, but the individual postures are beneficial as well. After learning all of the postures, refer to the sample routines in Chapter 6 for guidance on building a practice set.

Holding the sphere is a posture you may have seen before, but please read the entire description and instruction through anyway. There are likely details that are different that will be beneficial.

1. Stand in the Horse stance with your feet shoulder-width apart. (Use the same steps as mentioned earlier.)

2. Inhale and let your arms rise with your breath. They should feel as though they are floating up in water.

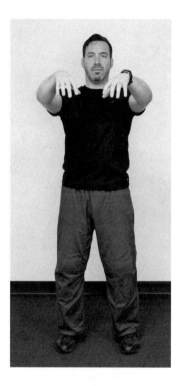

3. Let your arms create a circle as if you are holding a large sphere in front of your chest. (Imagine a large ball or sphere.) Some people say it looks like you are hugging a tree, and it does to a certain degree.

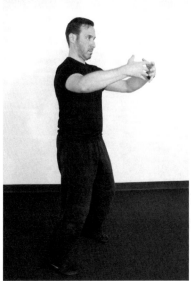
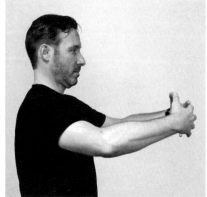
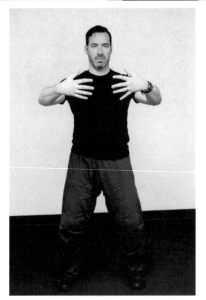

4. Relax into the stance, but be mindful of the form. This is the crux of all standing. Relax your muscles, but keep the form. Your muscles are neither stiff nor slack but somewhere in between.

5. Take an inventory to maintain the stance. Start with making sure your head is floating up. Imagine a string tied to the back of your head which will make your head straight.

6. Imagine there is a pole going through the center of your body, and it keeps your body straight without being tense. You are in alignment from your feet to the top of your head.

7. Keep your shoulders relaxed and your knees slightly bent.

8. Breathe deeply. Try the counting method described earlier.

This stance is a great overall energy boost, but it is also the foundation for everything that will follow. If you had only moments to practice one stance, this would be the one to do. You will feel an overall sense of well-being and a raised energy level, as well as a better sense of balance.

As you stand, remind yourself of a few things: be sure to think of your head floating up, the pole going through your body, and your arms floating as if in water. You will also need to remind yourself to let your shoulders drop. Use a mirror to check these details. To ensure you don't build any bad habits, be sure to check yourself both straight on and sideways in the mirror.

Holding the sphere below

1. Imagine you are holding a sphere about the size of a basketball in front of you. It should be about the level of your navel. Let your hands wrap around the ball and become rounded. Be sure to keep the palms facing each other.

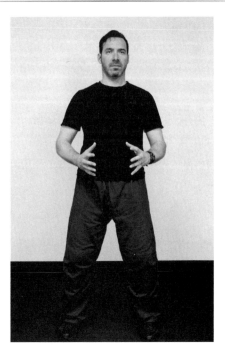

2. The steps are the same for this posture as for the previous one.

3. Imagine there is a beam of light going between the two palms.

4. As you breathe feel the palms slightly move away from each other as you inhale, and then move back as you exhale. Sometimes the feeling of the two palms has been compared to two magnets resisting each other.

5. The benefits of this stance are especially specific to the hands and arms. If you have any hand issues, try standing in the stance for 15–20 minutes each day and you may feel some positive effects.

This posture is the one that my friend was given by a TCM doctor to help him with arthritis in his hands. It is a great posture to improve the hands. There was a time when I was working on a computer for up to 70 plus hours a week and I always used this posture daily for about 5 minutes a day. It seemed to make my hands feel better. I probably should have developed carpal tunnel syndrome, but I never did. My hands felt great and still do.

Often you will feel energy between your hands, and they will feel as if they are repelling each other like two magnets. When I feel good, the energy is stronger, and when I am feeling ill, it is weaker. See what *you* feel. Try it out.

Holding the sphere away

1. The stance for your legs is the same: Horse stance.

2. Let your arms float up and feel as though you are pushing a sphere away from your face. Your hands will be rounded and your intention is as if you are pushing something away from you. Your hands should float to face level.

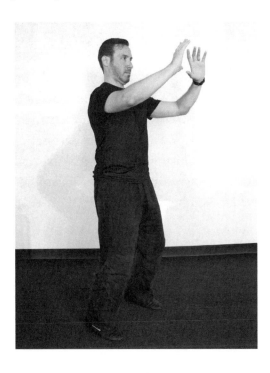

3. You should not lean forward. The feeling should be subtle and the stance should look the same as the others to an onlooker and when you check it in the mirror.

4. The thought that you are holding a sphere, and gently pushing away from it, is the main goal in this posture.

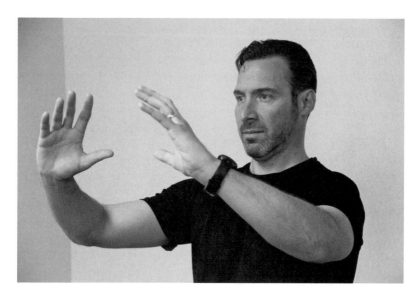

This posture is often the most challenging, as the shoulders may tend to rise. Check them and ensure that they are not rising. Relax and drop the shoulders. Don't exert more muscular strength in the arms to keep your arms up than is necessary. Continue to think of your arms as floating up. This may be challenging, but it is not insurmountable. With continued focus and practice you will feel relaxed as you hold the posture.

Holding the sphere down

1. Let your arms float down and imagine the sphere is trying to rise. With your mind you are gently holding the sphere down.

2. Your hands should be about the same level as your navel.

3. Be careful not to lean forward. Remember that the mental directives are subtleties that you will feel but not see.

4. The rest of the posture is the same as the previous ones.

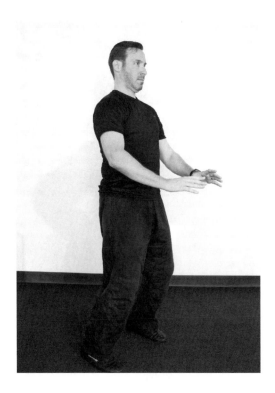

This posture is often very calming. Try to feel the sphere rising as you gently hold the sphere down. The emphasis is gentle. Don't exert external force. The feeling should be pleasant and calm. Imagine a balloon trying to rise and you gently hold it in place. Once again, retain the upright posture. Check yourself in the mirror and make sure that you are not leaning forward.

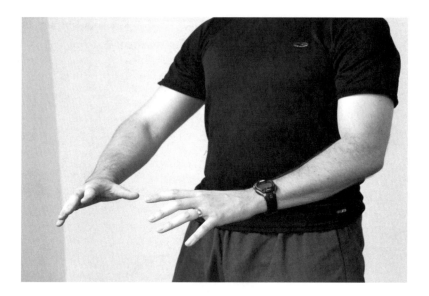

Holding the sphere from behind

1. Let your hands gently float to your back at about kidney level. The back of your hands rest against your kidney area.

2. Imagine the sphere is behind you, and that you are gently pushing the sphere behind you.

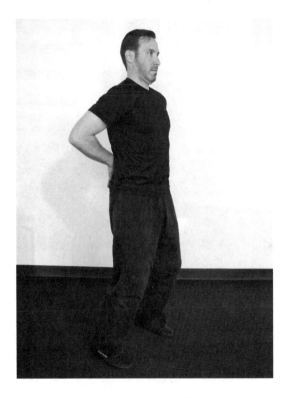

3. The most common error with this form is raising the shoulders to move the hands, so move very slowly and drop your shoulders before you start.

4. You should check with a mirror to be sure that you are not raising your shoulders.

5. The rest of the posture is the same as the previous ones.

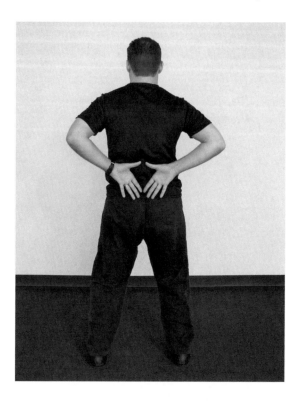

This posture rounds out the health postures. The hands and arms may seem as though they are in an odd position, but with some practice, you will find that the arms begin to feel more natural. Think of your arms in terms of curves instead of bending at the elbows or wrists.

You will be shifting your intention to your back so that you have a multidirectional shift included in your practice. Re-read the section on "Intention and awareness" earlier in this chapter to be sure that you understand the concept, as it may be new to you.

Feelings and changes

The first time you try the postures, I recommend doing one a day for a few minutes. Then you can start to add the other postures together and do them as a set. Start at 1 or 2 minutes each, if you can, and then gradually increase the time for each posture. As you become more proficient you will want to bend your legs a little lower and increase the time a little longer. Don't try to do both at once, though. You should either increase the time you are standing *or* try to bend your legs a little lower.

Be sure and be diligent, especially when getting started, to check your postures to ensure you are doing them correctly. Gradually, your body will start to acclimate to the postures. Initially, as with any form of exercise, your muscles will get sore, but they will get stronger, and you will perspire a bit as your temperature rises. This is normal. You should always remember that standing is *exercise*. It is meditative, which is different from most external exercises, but standing is definitely rigorous. With continued practice your body will get used to bending your legs and holding your arms in the various positions.

As your body adjusts and you lower your center of gravity a little, you will feel better balance and more stable. With continued practice you will notice that your arms hold the postures with little effort and yet feel strong. You can have your partner gently push against your arms as you hold the postures to ensure that you are using the internal directives, and not muscle, to maintain the postures.

As your body adjusts completely, and you are able to hold the postures with less effort, you will be able to add more of the visualization techniques. While you stand you will be exercising your body and mind together in a completely unique way which will benefit you for your whole life.

Part II

MARTIAL POSTURES

4

MARTIAL POSTURES

In traditional internal martial arts, such as Xing Yi Quan, Tai Chi Quan, and Ba Gua Quan, some form of internal or power training is taught. The student practices the forms for technique and the Qigong for power. One way to think of it is to imagine the techniques as a glass and the Qigong as the liquid that fills it.

As you read in the Introduction where I discussed my training in Xing Yi Quan, the San Ti Shi posture is of paramount importance. The best students that I know are diligent in practicing San Ti Shi. Perhaps coming from another martial art I benefited from the emphasis on power training. I already had many techniques and forms, and I was looking for the ingredient that would take power to the next level. For those who are not practitioners of martial arts, I would like to assure you that there is nothing contrary to a peaceful existence by studying martial arts or the martial postures. Often potential students come to me and say that they want to study something like Tai Chi Quan, but they don't want to study martial arts. People are always surprised when I tell them that Tai Chi Quan *is* a martial art. In Western thought we seem to misclassify what is a martial art and what is not.

Martial arts were developed for fighting, but studying them doesn't make the practitioner a hostile individual. In fact, most practitioners are incredibly peaceful. A person like myself, who came to martial arts through a tragedy, isn't looking for some kind of payback. The sense of empowerment and confidence an individual achieves tends to negate the need to prove oneself to others. Instead, students study as a meaningful lifelong pursuit of knowledge and as a means of keeping fit physically and mentally. This is sometimes referred to as the eternal student—always learning, so always gaining knowledge. As such, a person tends to be humble and slow to anger.

I hope that I am really making this clear so that you don't avoid the martial postures thinking that they may make you angry or agitated, or turn you into something you are not. Remember that they help cultivate energy, and that is their purpose. They can improve your health and make you feel more internal strength. Who doesn't want or couldn't use more strength and power? Try them out.

For martial arts practitioners, I can't tell you that you will turn into a comic book character, but you will likely feel a great sense of physical power when you practice the martial postures. As martial arts help to develop and require a healthy body, so these postures will help you with your health as well.

So why are these postures good for martial artists? Power. One of the purposes of the postures is to help practitioners feel rooted to the ground. By developing a strong root practitioners are able to better use their legs with driving power and are not able to be moved by their opponents easily. These are both tremendous advantages in a martial encounter. Practitioners will also feel that their arms can generate power more easily with less effort, and that they are using their whole body when moving. A feeling of almost effortless power is attained.

A strike with a relaxed arm from a strong posture with deliberate intention is very powerful. By practicing standing Qigong you will cultivate internal energy that is tangible. The longer you stand and the more often you practice, the more you will feel the difference. If you try it once and then try a punch, you will not notice anything. A sincere effort is required, and only a sincere effort will produce results. As you will notice in all of my instructions, consistency is the key.

The main physical difference between martial postures and health postures is that your weight should be slightly forward for martial postures. This technique will make the postures a little more challenging to hold, so you may want to start with your weight evenly distributed on your feet at first, and then, when you feel you are ready, you should shift your weight so that it is over the balls of your feet. Don't lift your heels high, though. The heels should basically be close enough to the ground that the shift is almost imperceptible. You should just be able to fit a piece of paper under the heels. If someone was watching you, they should not see a difference; however, you will definitely feel it. It is a subtle but powerful change.

As with all the standing postures, including the health postures, you can practice them individually and/or as a set. After a short period of time you should start to feel the benefits of the postures. Don't neglect the challenging ones, as that is how we grow. Simply start with a smaller amount of time and a greater amount of persistence.

Recently, with the popularity of mixed martial arts (MMA), traditional styles have suffered a negative backlash. As with all things, there are good and bad aspects. Some of the backlash is warranted, and some is not, just as some of the praise for one martial art as being superior to everything else is not correct for everyone. We seem to live in a world of extremes where there often can be no middle, and that is unfortunate. I know that there are some people who will discount the contents of this entire book without even trying it, because they have come to the erroneous assumption that there is nothing beyond the external, and that things like standing Qigong are some kind of weird mythology. One person told me that they don't believe in developing energy and intention, because they can't see it. I reminded them that you can't see air or electricity either, but you *can* see the effects of them. Likewise, there are others who have an unrealistic view of the internal that is something approaching magic. One teacher was offering to teach a "force field" that couldn't be punched through. That seemed like an extraordinary claim, and I think such claims harm people and reputations. I hope that practitioners of all arts will give standing Qigong a try, and not disregard it as hocus pocus that doesn't work. The postures may appear deceptively easy, but once they are tried I think the practitioner will agree they are suitably challenging for any martial arts practitioner, and they will provide a new dimension and depth to your training.

Ultimately, standing Qigong builds the mind-body connection. What martial artist can't benefit from that? I study Judo as well as traditional Chinese arts, and I have noticed that standing has helped me with a strong foundation. Some of the postures are especially beneficial. When fighting for grip or when throwing, it is preferable to get the strongest base you are able to. The "holding the sphere" posture helps develop the strong root that is used for both. The arm's soft yet powerful extension is cultivated in the San Ti Shi posture. The front-arm extension, relaxed but with intention, is great for keeping the opponent in position with a powerful grip. For the groundwork (ne-waza) I felt that the twisting motion of the Dragon posture (see later in this chapter), for example, provided a comfortable feeling for the odd positions one often finds themselves in on the ground. There are likely countless other associations that can be made when you study these postures and feel the benefits as you study your art.

I hope that I have convinced some skeptics (of which I used to be one) to at least try this traditional power training and see how it helps you with your chosen application. Regardless of whether you study an internal art, such as Tai Chi Quan, Ba Gua Quan, or Xing Yi Quan, or an external art, such as Karate, Judo, or MMA, you will feel the difference if you keep up with your standing practice.

Martial standing postures

The martial standing postures are as follows:

1. San Ti Shi

   ○ San Ti Shi (variation: holding the sphere)

2. Tiger

   ○ Tiger I

   ○ Tiger II

3. Rooster

   ○ Rooster I

   ○ Rooster II

4. Dragon

Follow the directions for each posture as closely as possible when first learning them. After you have a better understanding of them, go back and re-read the section on the posture you are using so that you can make sure you are getting all of the details to help you do it correctly. It may take a few readings in conjunction with your practice to make sure that you have it correct. As you notice the things that need to be adjusted, simply make the adjustments and avoid any negative feelings about previous practice mistakes. Always move forward.

San Ti Shi

San Ti Shi is the cornerstone of the art of Xing Yi Quan, so I think this is a good place to start for the martial postures. There are many variations on how the feet are weighted in the stance (50/50, 60/40, 80/20, and so forth), but I think that 50/50 is best. You can experiment with different weighting, but I think that you will find more benefit with the 50/50 weighting.

Having the legs weighted evenly is better for building a strong foundation for health and martial arts applications. In the other variations the back leg is the leg with more weight, and the front leg may be lighter.

Using a mirror for a side view and a frontal view will help you see that you are holding the posture correctly, but once you have ensured that it is correct, you should *feel* the posture as much as possible. Remember that the connection of your mind and body, and development of internal power, is what you are trying to cultivate, so the use of internal images and searching for the feeling is what you want to strive to achieve.

1. Stand with your feet together. Relax and breathe naturally and diaphragmatically.

2. Spread your arms widely, with your palms facing up.

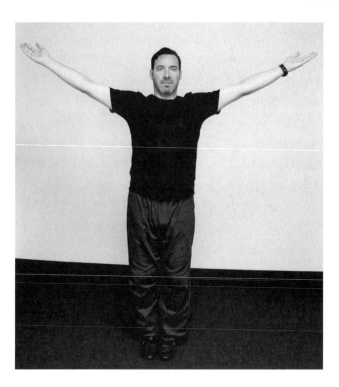

3. Move your arms above your head, with your elbows slightly bent, and palms facing each other.

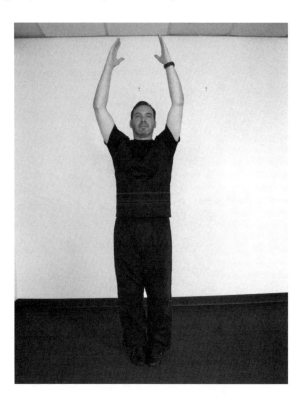

4. Make a big circle with your hands and bend your knees as you sink down. As the hands come together, they will come together as two fists facing each other.

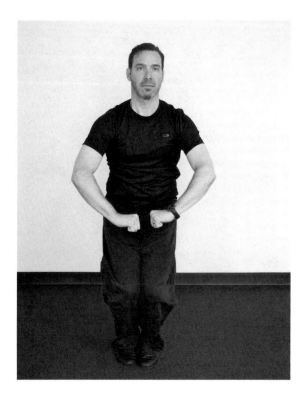

5. Drive your right hand out under your chin (as pictured below) and bring it to rest just below your navel (as in the photo on the next page). Step towards the direction you are punching with your left leg. (If you start at the 12 o'clock position, you should turn and end up in the 9 o'clock position.)

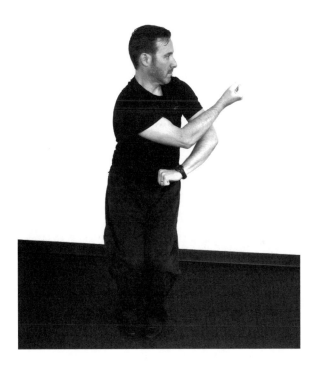

6. As your right hand comes to rest, raise your left hand up and away from you and bring it to rest in the position shown in the photo on the next page. Your two hands should move simultaneously in opposite directions. The hands and legs moving into position should look as if they are "unfolding" into the final posture.

7. As you stand in the posture, make sure that your feet are in the correct alignment. The right leg should be pointing at about a 45-degree angle, and the left leg should be pointing straight.

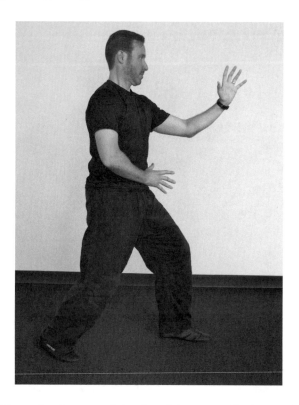

8. Keep the image of the head being pulled straight up in this posture as well. Relax the arms without making them weak. The arms should feel full of energy without feeling too stiff or slack. Imagine that the energy is shooting from your first finger and looping up and making a circuit through the top of your head.

9. The hands should have the intention of holding two small spheres. They should be neither flat nor too bent, but rounded.

10. Try the posture with your heels on the ground the same as in the health postures, then after some time, try shifting your weight to the balls of your feet. You will notice the increased stress on your quadricep muscles. Your heels will rise slightly (so slightly that another person won't really notice).

Treat this posture as the most important of the martial postures, as it is the best way to start incorporating more challenging ways of using your arms and legs while using the skills you learned in the health postures, such as diaphragmatic breathing and feeling your center.

San Ti Shi variation: holding the sphere

The San Ti Shi posture has a variation involving "holding the sphere" that is the same as the previous version with the exception that your arms look as though you are holding a sphere slightly to your side. Be sure to think of your arms as actually holding a sphere to keep the arms rounded.

1. The opening for this posture is the same as for San Ti Shi. Follow steps 1–6 from the previous posture.

2. Let your arms float up as if you are holding a sphere at your side. Your left palm should face your chest, and your right palm should face your left bicep.

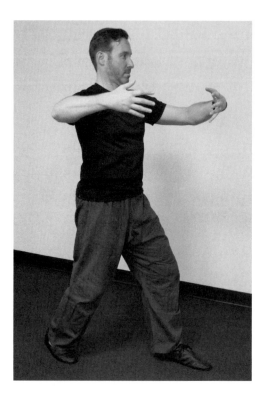

While standing in these postures be sure to take inventory of the physical requirements of the postures. Keep asking yourself questions to be sure you are in the right position. Once you have the physical posture in a good position, you can start using visual imagery.

You should feel strong but not tense. You can have a partner gently push against your body and arms to be sure that they are full of energy and not weak. Passive resistance should be used so that you can relax into the form of the posture without feeling tense. Resist without feeling like you are resisting. Words are difficult to adequately describe this feeling, but suffice to say it is relaxed with form and yet not limp. Think of energy flowing through your body. In the same way that the content of water flowing through a hose gives the hose expansive volume and makes the shape strong from its previous flaccid form, so does the feeling of relaxed energy flowing through your body.

Tiger

The next two postures are both called the Tiger. These forms are very rewarding once you start to feel them. As befitting the word *tiger*, they should generate a strong stable posture with similar energy.

Tiger I (Xing Yi Quan Tiger)

The first Tiger form is from Xing Yi Quan and is similar to San Ti Shi. The foundation is the same, but the arms are held in a different position. This posture will feel more active forward, but be careful not to lean.

In Xing Yi Quan there is a movement form based on this standing form. This form is excellent for developing energy to enhance your martial arts and promote vigorous health. This is a good form to transition to from San Ti Shi when you are standing in multiple forms in succession.

Preparation for Tiger I is the same as that for San Ti Shi (refer to previous San Ti Shi pictures).

1. Start extending your hands as if striking with the blade/ little-finger side of your hand. The palms of both hands face each other. (If you are looking at yourself in a mirror, your palms will frame your face.)

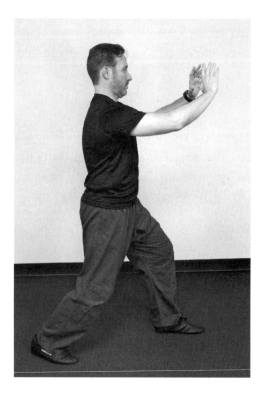

2. Be careful not to lean forward.

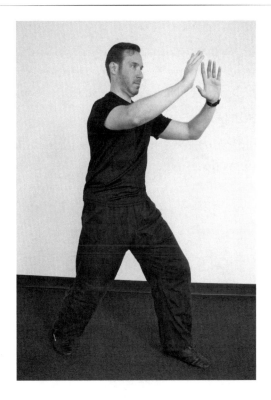

Your posture should feel strong driving forward. If you have your partner gently push against your hands, they should not give, but be resilient with only as much effort as is necessary. You should be active forward without leaning. Your body should be the same as in San Ti Shi.

As you go through your mental inventory while standing, pay particular attention to your shoulders. Be careful that they don't start to rise up. Most of us are quite tense and probably used to our shoulders rising up, but you will need to make an effort to drop your shoulders as you stand.

You can also turn your hands slightly outward and use the arm-and-hand position from the "holding the sphere away" posture that you learned in Chapter 3. The body, legs, and the rest of the posture will remain the same.

Tiger II

The second Tiger posture is from Yi Quan. Yi Quan is a great art that incorporates standing Qigong in a similar way as Xing Yi Quan for developing power. Follow the steps provided to attain the posture properly.

1. In preparation for standing in the posture, inhale and let your arms float up.

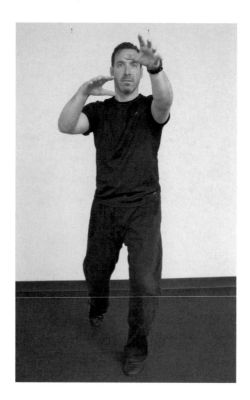

2. Step back right and sink down.

3. The arms rise and then settle down.

4. The feet should be in the form of an "L." The stance is deep, so drop as low as you can.

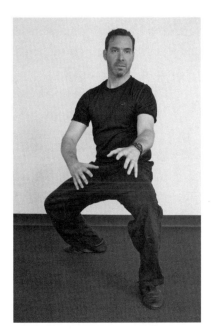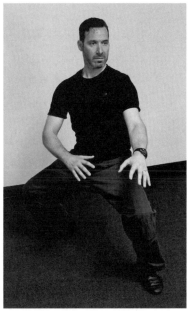

Once you start practicing the stance regularly you will want to try to stay lower longer. Relax your shoulders and arms. Let your upper body remain relaxed. Let your hands be slightly rounded. Breathe deeply and keep your upper body pressing up.

The Tiger stances are great for building up internal and physical strength quickly. You will develop a strong foundation and feel greater stability in your martial arts. Practicing both Tiger postures as a set is a good way to build more power. Be sure to practice on both sides.

Rooster

The rooster (sometimes called chicken) is not commonly considered a fighting animal in the West, but if you think of fighting roosters, you will better understand why it is deemed a fighting beast in martial arts and held in the same high esteem as the tiger, dragon, and serpent, for example.

The Rooster postures involve holding your posture on one leg. These postures will build better balance, leg strength, and internal power. The Rooster postures were the martial postures that I noticed provided the biggest change in myself. Within a very short time I felt my balance was better and my legs felt incredibly strong. These postures are challenging and rewarding. If you want to improve your martial arts, then be sure to include at least one of the Rooster forms in your practice routine.

Rooster I

The first Rooster form is from Xing Yi Quan. There are two Xing Yi Quan moving forms that include this posture. This posture embodies the essence of the form. Although both of your feet are on the ground, your weight should be almost entirely on one leg. The other foot should be barely touching the ground. Think of the foot as testing bath water. It has form but is not supporting your weight.

1. In preparation for the posture, relax and stand with your feet together.

2. Raise your right hand and shift your weight to your left leg.

3. Bend your right leg.

4. Your left hand should be by your side in a loose fist.

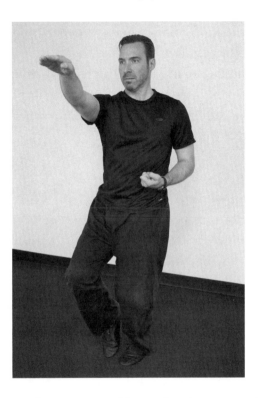

There are some things to consider and to be aware of when you practice this posture:

- Relax your extended right arm and only use as much energy as you need to keep your arm raised and extended.

- Drop your shoulders, especially on the arm that is extended.

- Sink into the posture, but keep your back straight and your head feeling as though it is floating up.

- The hand on the extended arm should be in front of you.

It may be easier to think of energy flowing through your extended arm and that is what keeps it extended. For the hand that is beside you, think of holding an egg in your hand. Be sure that you are not clenching the fist tightly. Your body and arms should be relaxed and feel comfortable. The leg that is supporting your body will feel your weight and will gradually be bent lower. Feel the leg getting stronger. Practice the posture on both sides for the same amount of time on each side.

Rooster II

The second Rooster posture is from the art of Yi Quan. This posture is similar to the previous Rooster posture in that it includes standing on one leg, but beyond that it is very different. This posture is excellent for building internal energy and martial power. Try to stand for longer periods of time gradually, and pay particular attention to your spine. Make sure the spine is straight.

The preparation for this posture is the same as previous postures in that you should stand still and relax. Breathe deeply and, when you are ready, start the movement for the posture.

1. Relax and feel as though you are stomping down onto your right leg as you drive up your left leg.

2. Let your arms float up. Your arms will be held as though they are holding a ball to your side. (The arms are the same as the variation of the San Ti Shi posture.) Be sure to drop your shoulders.

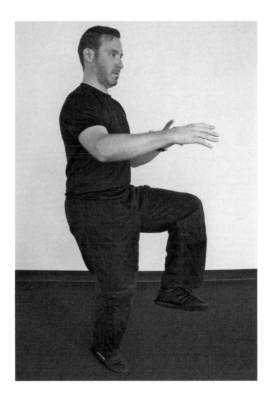

3. Hold up the leg with no tension and try to make it have a rounded feel like your arms. If you drop deeper on the leg you are standing on (the right leg in this case), you will feel greater stability. Initially, this will be challenging until you build up your leg strength, but you will benefit greatly over time.

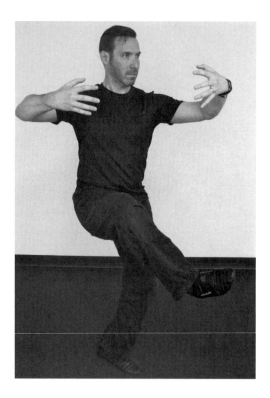

As with the first Rooster posture, stand for the same amount of time on both sides. Be sure to think about all of the basic points in all standing postures. Relax and use only as much energy as necessary. Let your head float up. When you stomp down, be sure to actually make a stomping motion slowly so that you transfer the weight correctly.

Balance is going to be an issue initially, and that is one of the great benefits of this posture. Your balance will be greatly improved, and your legs will become much stronger. Still, it is important to resist the urge to stand in the posture without following the guidelines we have been using so far. For example, if you stand in the posture and find yourself teetering unsteadily, go ahead and put your foot down for a moment, and try starting over with more emphasis on the principles.

As this is probably the most challenging posture in the book, you will want to treat it as such and take your time when gauging your progress. Use small amounts of time to start, and pay particular attention to the feeling you initially get when you stomp down on the supporting leg. If you are feeling balanced when you start, you will probably stay balanced as you stand. Likewise, if you are unbalanced and wobbling, you will likely not get the balance to resolve this.

This is a great posture for developing stronger throwing, such as in Judo, as well as kicking, such as in Kung Fu and Karate.

Dragon

The Dragon is a powerful posture, but it must be practiced carefully. This posture encompasses many of the attributes of the mythical Chinese dragon. As you will notice in Chinese art, the dragon's body is always depicted as twisting as it flies through the heavens with its arms and legs extended. The dragon represents the softer motion in martial arts, and the tiger represents the hard. In keeping with this philosophy you will want to be relaxed as you go through the preparation steps and ultimately as you hold the final posture.

As with all of the postures, be sure to use a mirror to check your form. The Dragon posture will build up your energy and leg strength as well as provide a more natural feeling to the twisting motion. The feeling of extension and twisting are essential to doing the posture correctly.

This form is from a style of Yi Quan, but as with all of the forms, practicing the Dragon will provide anyone with more internal energy and benefit any martial arts or Qigong practitioner. Follow the steps below to perform the posture.

1. Step out with your left leg and stand in San Ti Shi.

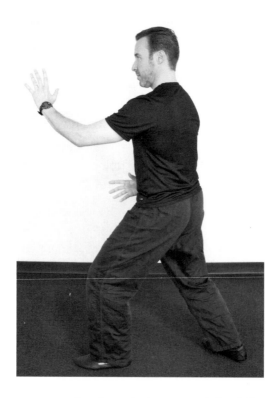

2. Let your arms begin twisting toward the left.

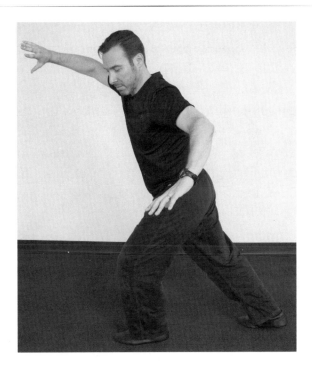

3. Pivot on the ball of your supporting foot. Look at your heel on the extended leg.

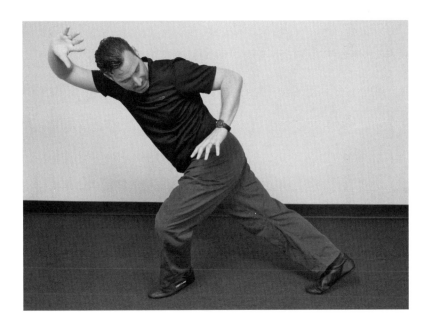

Your spine should feel as though you are extending, elongating, and twisting. Your hands should feel as though they are holding/pushing two balls. The left leg should be bent deep enough to support the body with stability.

The Dragon posture should feel as though you are pushing with your hands and elongating with your body all at the same time. As with all of the martial postures, practice the posture on both sides for the same amount of time. Gradually increase the length of time to make your practice more challenging and more rewarding.

This posture is good for styles that incorporate ground grappling, such as Judo, as well as styles that incorporate twisting, such as Ba Gua Quan.

When you first start standing in the postures, you will notice that your body feels the effects of standing, like in other forms of exercise. Your legs and shoulders will ache a bit as you start using these muscles and some other muscles that you didn't even know that you had. With continued practice you will acclimate quickly. Your body will get used to the demands made upon it and you will feel more comfortable. Gradually, you will use only the amount of energy required. Remember, as with anything you want to excel in, persistence and consistent practice is the key.

PART III

THE FIVE ELEMENT FORM

5

THE FIVE ELEMENT FORM

Although this book has focused on standing postures, I wanted to include a moving form so that you can feel the energy generated from standing postures incorporated with movement. In the internal art of Xing Yi Quan, the Five Element Form is very important. It is a method for cultivating energy as well as technique.

The five elements of Xing Yi Quan refer to the five individual element forms, their corresponding energy, and their relation to the organs of the human body in TCM. The five elements are wood, water, fire, metal, and earth. They correspond to the organs in the body in the same order as lungs, liver, kidneys, heart, and spleen. The characteristics of the elements are found in the individual elements. Theoretically, by practicing the five elements you are cultivating the various energies and practicing the individual motions in a form that, while not very long, will provide a thoughtful, rigorous, and internally powerful workout. With all of the motions of the five individual elements, many different permutations of the basic forms can be devised. You will notice that one of the motions is called "White Crane Spreads His Wings." Although the crane is not one of the twelve animals in Xing Yi, the crane is ubiquitous in Chinese martial arts and so it is included in the Five Element Linking Form.

The hands are shown in fists, but be sure not to keep your hands clenched into fists the whole time. You should relax your hands, and tighten into fists when you are showing a strike, and then let them relax again. Everything should be coordinated with the breath. Think of everything "arriving together." The breath, strike, and step all happen at once with your intention. That may be a lot to coordinate all at once, so you can try focusing on the breath and footwork first, and then start to concentrate on the hands, as they are the easiest to correct.

The simplicity of the form, as with all aspects of Xing Yi Quan, is its most attractive quality to me. There are no tricky angles, as the form is basically linear, which is a very prominent aspect of Xing Yi Quan. With the execution of the form you will be incorporating the alignment, breathing, and centerline that you learned in the standing postures. The form has very few postures and movements, so it can be learned fairly quickly. The form is usually done in a very explosive and powerful way as you transition from one position to the next, but it can also be done slowly and incorporate the same slow and steady motion associated with Tai Chi Quan. I often teach the form in the slow manner and it is best to do it slowly at first. The body, breath, and intention are the same; only the speed is different. Once you learn the form you should try it both fast and slow.

Description of the Five Element Form

The Five Element Form consists of two lines. You will move in one direction, then turn around and go in the other direction, and end up where you originally started. The stepping is done in either a full step or half step. The half step is sometimes called step and correct. A half step is done as a small step with the front foot, and the back foot adjusting behind, so that the feet are kept the same distance apart. In the half step, the back foot stays back, and the front step stays in the front. A full step is like walking: the back foot moves forward and the front foot moves back. Pay attention to the stepping patterns in the form as that will make understanding the form easier.

I would like to suggest a way that I think will make learning the form easier: I don't suggest trying to learn all of the various parts at once. I suggest learning one and then two parts, and then tying them together. Then learn the next part and practice those parts together. Focus on making each part correct, and then when you are satisfied, add the new part. If you use this method of building the form, you will have an easier time memorizing the form and understanding each part.

This is a good method for learning anything new, and I use it often. Start small and build onto what you have. Before long, you will be doing well and making progress. I first learned this method in music school and used it for learning long pieces and parts, and it worked really well. In addition to small steps, be sure to take breaks from it often and for short periods (just for a minute or two). Don't hammer on something for long periods without stopping. You will likely only get frustrated and not make much progress.

1. *Salute:* Open the form with the salute, and move to San Ti Shi. All Xing Yi Quan forms begin this way.

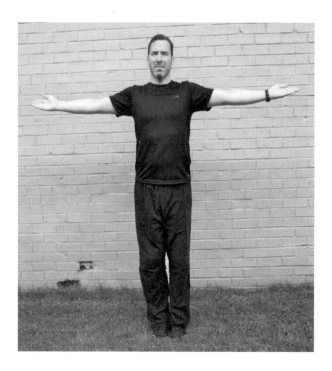

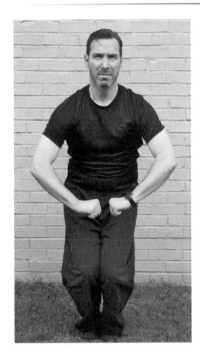

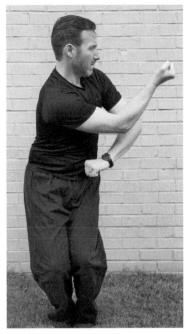

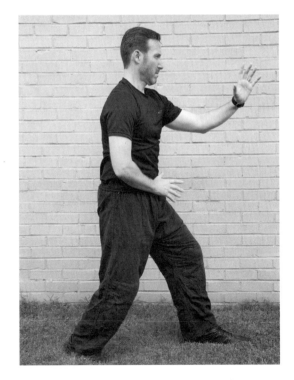

2. *Wood:* Make a small step forward with your left foot and correct with your right foot as you punch right. This is the element of wood. This stepping pattern is called half step.

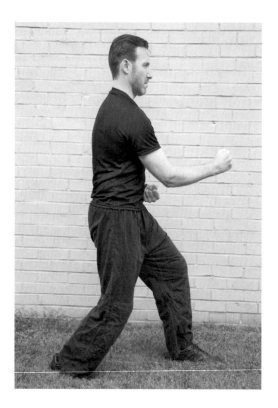

3. *Water:* Make a full step back with your left foot. Move your left hand up in front of you as your right hand moves down.

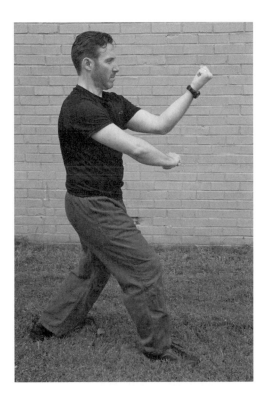

4. *Wood:* This version of Wood is the same as the first, just stepping with the right leg in the half step instead of the left. Note: the hands are the same. Let the left hand move in a circle down to your navel. Let the right hand move forward as pictured.

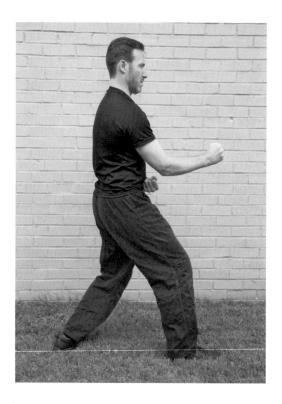

5. *White Crane Spreads His Wings:* Let your arms rise like you are stretching to yawn in the morning. The hands separate above your head. Then your right fist will strike your left palm as you step (if done slowly) or stomp (if done quickly) with your right foot.

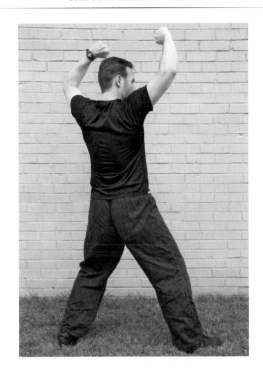

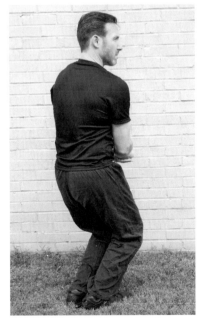
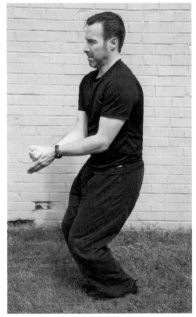

6. *Fire:* Raise your right hand over your hand as if blocking your head, and punch straight with your left hand. Make a full step right to 45 degrees. (If you were to use a clock face for reference, you would step to 2:00.)

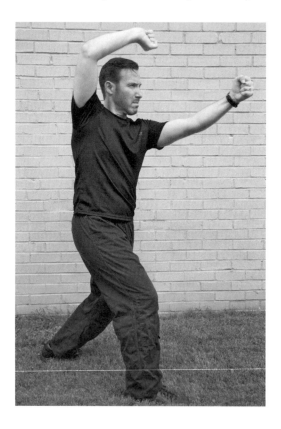

7. *Block:* Let your right arm cross your face with your wrist at eyebrow level. Let your left arm come to your side with your palm up.

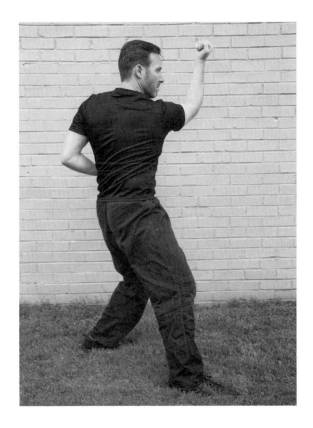

8. *Metal:* Let your left arm come up and forward in an arc or splitting motion as your right hand rests on your abdomen, as in San Ti Shi. Step back your right leg with a full step.

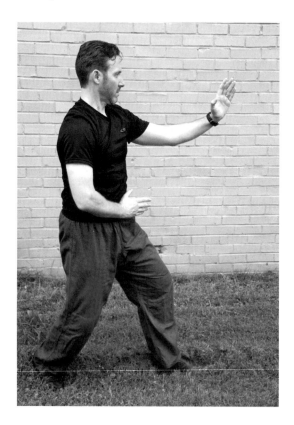

9. *Tiger Climbs the Tree:* Let your right arm and right leg rise, keeping the leg as straight as possible. It will be difficult to raise it very high at first, but as you practice it will become easier. It helps to think of the hand having a string tied to the leg which will bring the leg up when the hand goes up. (See image under step 13.)

10. *Tiger Climbs the Tree (continued):* The right hand draws down and the left hand moves forward with hands like claws (open hands). The right leg lands in cross step. (See image under step 14.)

11. *Wood:* Driving off your right leg, perform wood as in step 2. You should be left leg back and right leg forward before the turn.

12. *Turning:* This is the transition and turning technique. First bring your left hand to your abdomen next to your right hand, and turn on your left heel so that the toes are facing the right foot. (It should look roughly "pigeon toed.")

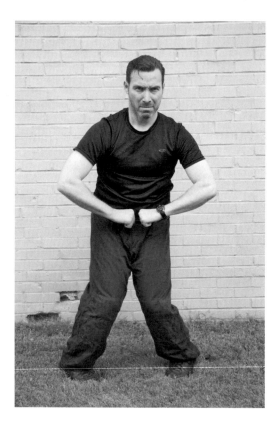

13. *Tiger Climbs the Tree:* Repeat step 9 facing the new direction.

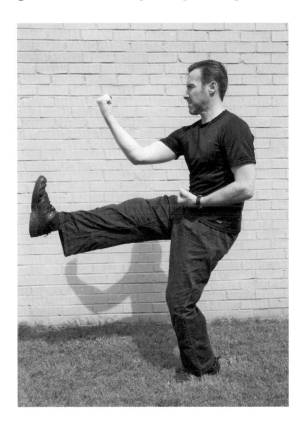

14. *Tiger Climbs the Tree (continued):* Repeat step 10.

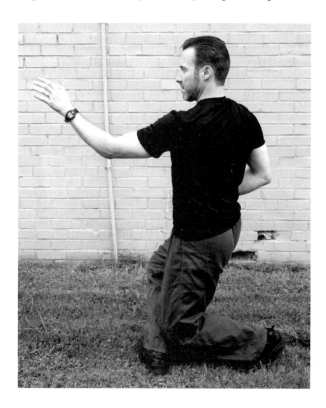

15. *Starting new line:* Driving off your right leg, you will begin the Wood element exactly the same as in step 2. The line will be exactly the same all the way to the "Tiger Climbs the Tree." Repeat everything up to step 15.

16. Repeat the lines as many times as you like up to 15 (Wood). To close, turn and do "Tiger Climbs the Tree" and "Wood" (steps 9 to 11) and, on the last line after Wood, add the final element: Earth.

17. *Earth:* Drive out with your left fist, and let the right fist come back to your abdomen. Step back with the left leg to cross step. The feel of the motion should be twisting. The hand goes forward as the hips twist.

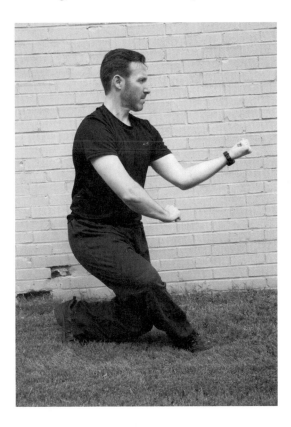

18. *End:* Bring the left foot to the right foot and salute to finish. See all the steps and note that you will rise to the same level where you began.

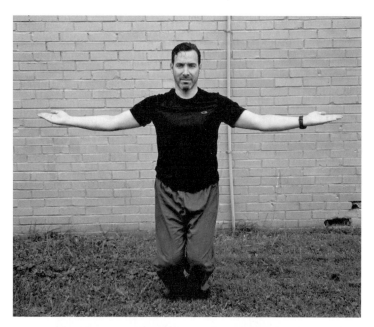

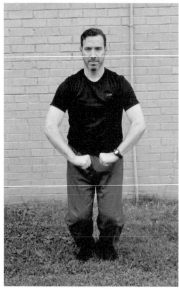

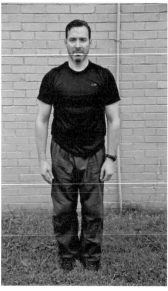

As mentioned previously, you can practice the form for as long as you want by simply not doing the last element of earth. You will truly benefit the most from doing several repetitions and then ending the form. It is common in Xing Yi Quan to do multiple repetitions for long periods. This process is called "running lines." As the form is short (only a few movements), repetition enables the practitioner to refine the technique of uniting the body, mind, and breath.

While you learn the form, pay particular attention to the footwork and then the hands. Be sure that when showing striking, your hands are in front of your body. That is the area where you have the most power. (If you need a refresher on alignment for the hands, refer to the "Alignment" section in Chapter 3, which talks about the "power zone.")

PART IV

DEVELOPING YOUR PRACTICE

6

PARTNER PRACTICE, SAMPLE ROUTINES, AND VISUALIZATION EXERCISES

Partner practice

Although standing Qigong is usually taught exclusively as an individual exercise, and that is usually how it is practiced, you can have a friend or fellow student help you improve your material. While practicing the postures you can have a partner to help you feel how you are progressing by having them check your posture's stability and also the feeling in your arms.

I learned about pushing against stances and postures to check for stability when I first started studying martial arts. I like to do the same with standing postures. It is a good way to feel if you are using your legs properly, staying in alignment, and also feeling your intention. The first thing to do is choose a posture. For ease of explanation, I choose holding the sphere, as it is the one you have probably been working with the longest. You can choose any posture. As you stand in the posture for several minutes, you can have your partner check your stability by having them gently place their hand on your shoulder from the front, and gradually and subtly increasing the amount of force they use.

As the person standing, the first reaction is usually to lean in the direction that you feel the force, but that would not be correct; instead, stay centered and shift your *awareness* to that direction. There will be subtle and imperceptible changes made in your posture, but all you have to do is remember to keep your center and be aware of the direction of force.

The next thing to do is have your partner do the same thing from your back. The next locations to move to are the sides of your shoulders. When completed, you will have shifted awareness to four directions (front, rear, both sides). This will help you feel your center and your intention as well. Be sure that your partner doesn't push too hard, especially when you try it the first time. It is important that you start with a little pressure at first and then gradually build from there. Be very cognizant of leaning. Make sure there is no lean.

Once you have tried stabilizing the body, you can move to the arms. The arms will really require some visualization. As you hold the sphere, have your partner gently push on your forearm. The first reaction is usually to resist with your muscles. Instead of trying to resist your partner's force with force, try to think about your arms being full of energy. You can think of energy surging through the arms, making a circuit through the gaps between your hands and feeling powerful.

As with the partnered stability exercise, make sure you have a good feeling and have been standing for a few minutes before you try adding pressure. You can use this method for all of the postures, whether for health or martial arts, to help you develop a strong foundation and awareness of your body. This exercise will also give you a tangible way of feeling how you are developing.

Choosing the right partner may be the most important part. Be sure that your partner is someone that truly wants you to succeed and is interested in what you are doing. Often people, such as friends and family, although seemingly well meaning, can sabotage our success. In my classes I usually have people who are only casual acquaintances work with each other, as you tend to get a more honest effort and sincere cooperation from both people.

Sample routines

The sample routines below are a way for you to get started, but they are merely my suggestions. As you practice you will want to modify your practice to better suit your needs by adding time and details such as bending lower. You will also want to experiment with mixing different postures and creating your own practice sequences or merely honing in on one posture that you want to perfect or that provides you with something that you want. An example would be to use the Tiger postures to build up your legs or the Rooster forms for balance.

As a general rule, you should strive to stand longer and lower, but don't try to accomplish both things at once. Either stand with a lower stance or stand for a longer duration.

When you are practicing, you should first focus on good form. Once you have the form correct take an inventory of your body by asking yourself the following questions: Are you relaxed? Are you breathing from your diaphragm? Are you dropping your shoulders? Once you have these items mastered you can move on to using imagery to help you maintain the postures, such as holding the sphere and visualizing the sphere as a source of energy.

The secret to attaining results is not how long you stand, but how often. It is not standing for 30 minutes once a week, but rather standing for a few minutes every day. It is consistency that will make the difference. If you have only 5 minutes one day, then stand for 5 minutes. You will discover that you can find more time than you thought when you don't eliminate standing practice all together. As busy as we all are, we can find the time if we make it a priority. Start now and keep at it.

Routine I

1. Holding the sphere

Practice holding the sphere for 5 minutes. You can start with a lower amount of time if necessary, but add time at about 30 or 60 seconds a day. Once you can stand for 5–10 minutes, try bending your legs a little lower for the same amount of time.

Routine II

When practicing the following routines, hold each posture for 1 minute:

1. Holding the sphere

2. Holding the sphere below

3. Holding the sphere away

4. Holding the sphere down

5. Holding the sphere from behind

Use the same guidelines as in Routine I. This is a set that will really enhance your health, so the sooner you can work it in, the better. You should feel great after you do it. Don't forget to start increasing the time for each posture as you progress.

Routine III

1. Rooster II (1 minute for each leg)

2. San Ti Shi (5 minutes for each side, right and left)

3. Holding the sphere

This set is a good way to ease into the martial stances. Try to add time to the Rooster stance quickly, and you will feel the effect on your martial arts with better balance and stability. If you feel that you are able to increase the length of time quicker than I have suggested, then by all means you should do so. If you feel that you want to do more, then do more.

The holding the sphere posture is a good way to think about consolidating your health and energy into your body. Try alternating with one of the other health postures as well.

Routine IV

1. Tiger II (1 minute for each side)

2. Rooster II (1 minute for each leg)

3. Holding the sphere

Use the same guidelines as in Routine III.

Routine V

1. Holding the sphere below (5 minutes)

2. Dragon (1 minute on each side)

3. Holding the sphere (5 minutes)

At first glance some people will likely be curious about the times, but I urge you to remember that you need to start small so that you actually start at all. As a teacher I have seen all too often where a well-meaning student comes every day for about two weeks and then I never see them again. Think of approaching these routines the same as eating. It is better to take small bites and chew slowly than to gobble down a large amount of food and choke.

I hope that these sample routines will show you the value of incorporating martial and health stances together. Create a sixth routine by choosing two martial stances and two health stances, and determine how long you will stand in each.

Experiment with different combinations and change your practice periodically for different purposes. As I mentioned previously, when I was concerned about my hands I used the holding the sphere below posture exclusively to make sure my hands were not damaged. When I am sick I use the holding the sphere posture for a short period of time. When I feel that I need to pump up my martial energy and train for more power I use the Tiger and Dragon postures. With such a variety of choices you can achieve the results you desire.

Visualization exercises

I have found the exercises below to be tremendously powerful when included with your standing Qigong practice as well as when used by themselves. The only caution that I have is to make sure that you are performing the postures correctly before you incorporate the additional visualization exercises. For some students it may take a few days, for some a few weeks, and for some a few months to get to the point where you can feel comfortable enough with the postures to incorporate visualization. It all depends on the person. Just remember not to rush it, and make sure your form is correct first. If visualization is completely new to you, you may want to try the visualization exercises on their own before you use the postures. The visualization techniques will still be effective, but when combined with your Qigong, you will feel the full benefit.

Exercise 1

In the instructions there is use of some visualization to get you into the posture, but with this exercise you can enhance the grounded (also called "rooting") feeling that you get while standing in a posture.

While standing, think of the space deep below your feet. Feel that there are long stakes coming from the bottoms of your feet, and that as you stand, they sink deeper into the ground. Visualize the stakes coming from your feet and penetrating several feet into the ground. Imagine that the stakes are made of a metal material and they are pointed with the tip buried deep in the earth.

Alternatively, imagine roots, as from a large tree, growing from your feet and reaching deep into the ground. Picture the thick twisting roots coiling in the earth like two large snakes reaching further and further down.

You may feel that your legs want to bend a bit deeper, and that is good. This is a great exercise for creating a stronger sense of rooting or grounding while standing. As you practice you will start to notice that you feel more "solid." When things become a feeling, that is when you are making the most progress.

Exercise 2

My friend was prescribed this exercise to treat his arthritis, and I really think this is one that everyone should try. Most of us spend a considerable amount of time working with computers, and often we don't take a break. All of us are susceptible to repetitive injuries, and I have found that this exercise is one of the best for preventing injury by creating awareness and having you focus on the hands. I used to work about 70 hours a week for a few years primarily on a computer, and I believe using this posture helped prevent me from developing repetitive injury to my hands.

It will work best in the holding the sphere below posture, although it can be used in others as well. While you stand and imagine the sphere, think of it as having a beam of energy going between your palms. As you breathe you can imagine this energy pulsing with your breath and making your hands warm and glowing with energy. Imagine that the energy makes your hands feel good, and relieves soreness and stiffness. As you breathe the hands get warmer and brighter with each inhale, and as you exhale they dim slightly. As you inhale the hands feel the energy expanding and making them separate slightly. With each exhale they feel drawn together.

Try to do this every day for a few days and weeks, and see how your hands feel. If you augment this exercise with Baoding health balls, you will help move things along. I use health balls, and I think they are a cheap and beneficial way to exercise your hands.

Exercise 3

Judging by the plethora of energy products on the market, having more energy is a pretty common desire for most of us. At my school most people have multiple jobs plus they are raising kids, so I understand that raising one's energy level is something we all would like to do.

This exercise is very good for raising or increasing energy. You can use it before a big event if you are a martial artist or a person with chronic fatigue. Even if you are just one of the millions of people who find contemporary Western culture exhausting, the exercise will work for you.

This exercise can be done in any posture, but for ease when beginning, you may want to try the first health posture: holding the sphere. As you stand, visualize energy in the form of yellow or white light coming through the bottom of your feet. The level increases through your legs, up to your hips, past your hips to your chest, and down through your arms to your fingers. The energy continues to rise until it reaches the top of your head.

Once you are "full of energy" you can imagine you are powered up. If you look at a phone or electronic device charging for reference, you can follow the same type of visual pattern. Once powered up, make sure it lasts for as long as you need it by merely thinking so. This is a great exercise and one I use quite a bit in classes and for myself. I have many different obligations, and any extra energy helps. Try it and see what you feel.

Exercise 4

I want to expand upon the example I gave earlier about using visualization for anxiety. Anxiety and all associated ailments and symptoms, such as fear and fatigue, are often the reasons students give me for wanting to study internal arts of any kind. Like diaphragmatic breathing, most people need more than just being told to "do it"—they need to be taught *how* to do it. One way to work with these feelings is through the way I suggested earlier, which is to visualize yourself doing something that you feel good and confident about. But what if you don't have anything you feel good about? What if you are so riddled with these feelings that you literally don't know what to do? You can try the exercise, but substitute yourself doing the things you want to accomplish as you would like them to be.

From my own experience I can tell you that I use this quite a bit as well. I work alone and do many different things. Many people depend on me, and if I can't complete tasks that are required, it will impact myself and others. I will pick something that probably happens to most people: driving to a location you have never been before. Sometimes there is the added pressure of a time constraint as well. So if the issue is going to a place you have never been before and you need to get there quickly, try this exercise.

Stand in any of the health postures and relax. As you stand, breathe deeply. Eventually, when you are in your posture for a few minutes and have the form correct, try using visualization. See yourself happy and in a relaxed state getting into the car. You feel confident because you have already looked up the location, so you have a map on your phone or car GPS, but regardless, you know that you will get there on time. You see yourself relaxed behind the wheel pulling out from where your car is parked, and easily merging onto the various streets. If there is a freeway, you see the cars pull into another lane to make room for you, and you thank them as you pull onto the freeway.

You see yourself doing what you normally do in your car. You listen to music or the radio. You see yourself at ease and traveling the same as if you were going to a place you have been many times. When you travel you are relaxed. You effortlessly pull up to the location and there is a parking spot for you within an easy trek to the front of the location. You exit the car feeling great and thinking about how wonderful the event you are attending will be. If you put an effort into this exercise, I believe that you will arrive in a better state than you would normally. Try it. What have you got to lose?

Exercise 5

This exercise should be practiced if you are finding it difficult to visualize. Think of it as a tutorial on using your mind and body together. I use this exercise when my students tell me that they find a particular exercise too difficult, or if they are just new to the whole idea of visualization. I am always surprised by how many people have never done any visualization at all. If this sounds like you, give it a try. Even if you are great at visualizing, try it out and it will improve your focus.

In the health stances we refer to the position of the sphere. You can take any of the exercises that utilize the sphere and follow these instructions. While holding the posture of your choice, picture the sphere as a red ball. Hold this image for a few moments and then picture it changing to a blue ball. As with the previous step, hold the image and now see the ball as glowing with positive energy. Hold this image for as long as possible. Now see the ball as red again.

Repeat the same process a few times. Then try using other colors or holding one image for a very long time. This exercise is great, and I think you will be surprised at how it affects your focus and concentration.

7

CONCLUSION

This book contains a great deal of material, but it is my hope that you did not find it too overwhelming. Take your time going through the postures and exercises and really feel comfortable with each of them before moving on. This is not the type of book you read once and set down, but rather a manual that you will hopefully refer to often. Sometimes, even with the best explanation and pictures, things can be missed, so re-read the sections you are focusing on to get the most out of them.

Practicing standing Qigong is contradictory to most of our often fast-paced lifestyles, so it will undoubtedly be unusual to accept a form of exercise with no motion, and yet it is a very beneficial form of physical and internal development. Even today people who have known me for some time, and know that I practice Qigong, are still skeptical about it. They sometimes ask me if I really do it or if I really "believe in it." My answer is always that I do practice, and it doesn't require belief, just sincere and patient practice.

As I mentioned when discussing energy, most people, particularly in the West, are prone to thinking of the body as a machine. I suppose it could be a leftover association from the industrial revolution, but although the body is an amazing piece of nature's engineering, it is more than just a machine. The elements as well as our emotions absolutely correspond and affect the body. Emotions can affect the body profoundly.

Emotions and health

I had never put much stock in the belief that emotions affect a person's health—until they affected mine. There was a time in my life when I was going through an issue that made me incredibly angry and anxious for a long time. I didn't notice it, but others certainly did. As I became more and more angry, it began to feel natural to be in this state.

I went to a doctor for a routine blood test and the results were quite unusual. I seemed to be in good health, but my liver enzymes were elevated. They were elevated enough to cause concern. The doctor wanted to do another blood test, so about a month later we did it again. My results were higher. I was getting a little concerned myself now. The doctor had me go in for an ultrasound.

I watched as the technician performed the ultrasound, and although they aren't supposed to tell you anything, you can usually tell what they think about what they are seeing. I asked some leading questions to no avail, but I didn't see any concern either, so I thought it was probably going to come out as negative for any problems. It did. At that point we (the doctor, the nurses, and myself) were all puzzled. What was going on?

The doctor said that they would try one more test. If the test came back the same or higher, they would have to perform a biopsy to see what was going on with my liver. I was extraordinarily concerned. I had difficulty thinking of anything else, but eventually I just resigned myself that this was out of my hands, and I would just have to see what happened.

I went in for the last test and I was pretty nervous about it. Did I have cancer? I had been quite a drinker before all of this, and I feared the worst. I had a pretty sleepless night over it. In the morning I called for the results and they said that they would have to mail them to me. I had to wait a couple more days. When the envelope arrived, I paused for a bit before opening it. I wanted to know, but I really didn't want to read it. I finally opened it up. The doctor had written across the results in big blue ink, *Looks good. No need for further tests.* I practically fell over with relief. But now I was puzzled. What had happened?

I spoke to my friend, who is a TCM doctor, and he asked what was going on in my life. I told him about the issue I was dealing with, and that it was something that definitely frustrated me. He asked if anything had changed before the last test, and I told him that in the interim before the last test, the situation which had caused so much stress and anger had been resolved. He said, "That's it." I was still confused. He told me that the emotion of anger is linked to the liver. I was stunned that I was letting my anger literally make me sick. Had it gone on, I could have done some damage to myself.

At that moment I made a real commitment to never let my emotions go unchecked again. The standing postures are one way that I center my mind and body. I have told this story to many people, especially when they discount the effects of stress. We have to take a few moments to calm down and get a hold of ourselves. Most of us live with levels of stress, anger, and fear that are probably doing us damage. We need to find ways to relieve ourselves. Standing Qigong is one constructive way to relieve stress.

Finding a teacher

I wrote earlier about finding a teacher, but what do you do if there is no Chinatown near where you live? Luckily, there are teachers in many places. When I moved to Georgia, I went looking for a new teacher at one point, and I found a few that I could study with, based on what I wanted to learn. I think you should have some criteria for a teacher, though everyone's criteria may be a little different.

My best friend and I studied Xing Yi Quan with the same teacher, but eventually he went to another teacher. Where I was looking for someone with a nice disposition and a lot of knowledge, he was looking for someone with a more robust personality. In the end we were both happy because we really knew what we wanted. I want to share with you some things that you can keep in mind when looking for a teacher that are not to be left to preference. Consider these the basic questions to ask for your search.

Does the teacher teach what you want to learn? This sounds like a pretty obvious question, but I routinely talk to people who study with people because they have heard that they are good, or that they should learn from them, but they really don't want to learn what they are teaching, and they may not even particularly like the way they teach. Ask yourself, "Do I know what I want to learn?" Are you looking to learn a fighting system? To study standing postures for health? Do you want to develop the ability to shoot lightning out of your hands? (Don't go to anyone who promises this one!) Think about what you want. Most of my students study with me to combat stress, or for health reasons. There are quite a few things that I can show them to help with these issues. I always ask my students what they want to achieve so that I can be sure I can help them. Make sure the teacher is teaching what is in alignment with your goals.

The next important factor is the location of your teacher. Is this teacher located someplace where you will go to learn on a regular basis? If they are too far away, it can be a convenient excuse not to study. As you have read previously, set yourself up for success and not failure. Make sure that you can make it to your lessons. It seems like an easy thing to consider, but I have found that location is important. I found a great teacher, but I couldn't make it to see him very often, so I looked for one closer, and I was able to be much more consistent.

When considering the location, you may want to think about all of the technical options that are available now. Things have changed with the internet, so there are many options available online now through certain communication tools, such as Skype, that were not possible before. (I have some students who travel quite a bit, and we have used Skype for lessons.) Some students don't like the online option and prefer to have the teacher with them in the same space, and although that is the best way, it is always an option to use the internet for people who are separated by a wide distance. If someone in Australia wants to study with me, for example, I would hope to use something like Skype to teach them.

Judge the teacher by what you experience, but also by their students. A lot of students are not necessarily an endorsement of great teaching, and having few students is not necessarily an indication of failure. There can always be other factors at work. Judge by how the students react to the teacher. Does the teacher want you to come study with him or her? Is he or she willing to help you if you have a question? What kind of feeling do you get? I am a pretty informal teacher, and some people like that, whereas others do not. I try to foster a community spirit in the school, and always welcome and introduce new people. Does the teacher have some students that he or she has been working with for a long time? Do they seem like they have some skill? As with most things that are new, go for the overall impression. If it is in line with what you are looking for, then start right away.

After years of teaching and being a student, I think that these issues are all worthy of consideration, and I am surprised when they don't come up very often. Don't take your training lightly. If it is worth your time, then it is worth some investigating to make sure that you make a good choice. I would hate to think that someone put little thought into having me teach them, when I put so much into being a good teacher.

Resilience

I can't emphasize enough the idea of starting right away. I hope this isn't too far off the beaten path in terms of the content of this book, but I feel it is necessary to address a very real concern for anyone starting anything new: procrastination—that insidious state of putting things off until they slowly dissolve into the easily justified excuse of not having enough time, and then we often simply quit all together. We do have the time, but often we make poor use of it. We simply need to make better use of our time. How long are we spending on Facebook to see what innocuous things people we don't really know anymore are doing? I spoke a little about this topic earlier, but I want to make sure that on top of learning about the subject of this book—standing Qigong— the reader realizes that the beginning of any new endeavor is so important that *how* you begin usually determines success or failure. I wanted to prove this to myself once, so I tried a project that I figured wouldn't amount to much, but it wound up being something very meaningful.

My project was to finish reading all of the books I had started in the previous year. After such a big buildup, you may think that this example is not particularly significant, but I hope you will stick with it. With this example I hope to prove my method and overall message about *how* you study something, which I think is at least as important as *what* you choose to study. I have always been a voracious reader and usually had the discipline to not start a new book until I finished another, but I had recently really fallen into a finicky state where I would start, say, a science book, then get bored with it, and then read a novel. Eventually, I would get bored with the novel and move to some kind of spirituality book and then to a slew of graphic novels (I am a fan of superhero comics); then I would see a movie and want to read the book, presumably so that I could say, "You know, the book was better than the movie." I guess none of us are above such things!

My nightstand had become stacked with books, to the point that it looked like a loosely organized free-form modern architecture exhibit. Each book had a piece of torn paper being used as a bookmark. Some bookmarks were well into the text and others just passed the author's preface or a foreword that had inexplicably stopped me cold. I was really ashamed by my lack of tenacity, and I felt that I was becoming what I had always feared: a quitter.

This example may seem extreme, using this unfinished-book anecdote to illustrate my point, but I have always felt that a person doesn't wake up one day and decide to become a quitter. We start by quitting a small amount, and then it builds up until we start to quit larger and more important things. My excuses were a litany of the modern ones that are used by most adults. You are undoubtedly familiar with them—excuses like "I am too busy" or "I need to do something for the kids." (I really don't even need to list them, as you are probably thinking of some right now!) We all seem to fall into this state.

I felt that the stack of books was knowledge outside of my head that was never going to enter without some real changes. It was also symbolic of what was going on inside myself. This was my moment of decision. Either I would change or continue as I had been doing. I started by putting all of the books in a box, and I started reading them for about 15 minutes a day. Even though I was reading one book at a time, I kept all of the books in the box with me wherever I read them. I read at the same time every day. In a few days I finished the first book and put it on a shelf. I picked up the next one and did the same thing. Eventually, I increased the reading time to 30 minutes as I was really enjoying this time spent reading. The books were slowly moving out of the box and onto the completion shelf. One by one they appeared on the shelf and the box got lighter until it was empty.

I felt pretty good about emptying the box of incomplete reads, and I was surprised that I hadn't done it sooner. Why hadn't I? I love to read. I had simply given up easily and succumbed to the modern malaise that seems to permeate our existence. At times we are resilient and can resist by shifting our focus, but sometimes we need to be brutally honest with ourselves and confront our nature, and see things as they are. I can't say that I never did this again, because I did, but I used the same method to make things right again. My message to my students, and the discipline I hold myself to in the various pursuits in which *I* am a student, is to start now. Start where you are and keep moving forward.

My hope for you

I commend you because you bought this book and read it, so hopefully you will now start a new chapter in your life with standing Qigong. This may have been a completely new experience for you, and soon it will be something you do every day and enjoy. What next? If this book has piqued your interest in martial arts, Qigong, meditation, or just new experiences in general, then I encourage you to continue. Challenge yourself and enjoy the new experiences you have. I never thought that I wanted to study martial arts, Qigong, or any of the things in this book, but one day I stepped outside my comfort zone, tried something new, and found a new path in my life. I hope you will do the same.